# Kindie Kung Fu

By William Gentry

Copyright © 2013 William Gentry

For Print versions:

ISBN-13: 978-1484895504

ISBN-10: 1484895509

For e-book versions:

ISBN: 9781301504220

# Table Of Contents

## Acknowledgements

Master Jeffrey Noel Reader; my Tae Kwon Do and Ju jitsu instructor from OKC

*Shifu Rick Krause, Shifu Peter Shumway, Shifu Wei Lun Huang my Tai Ji instructors from OKC, Wang *Laoshi from China, Jian Laoshi from Taiwan; my *Neijia instructors, Mr. Lin my *Shui Jiao instructor from Taiwan

*Shifu=Master Worker

*Laoshi=Teacher

*Neijia=Internal Martial Arts

*Shui Jiao=Chinese Wrestling

******

## Dedication

To my mom and brother, thanks for believing in me, I love you both

******

## Special Thanks

To all the people at my kindergarten. Especially; Vicky, Herman, Emily, Lillian, Terrence and Yoyo! To mi amor, Paola. Much Love and Thanks.

## About the Author

My journey into the world of martial arts began at age 6 when I first saw "The Karate Kid." I did my best imitations of martial arts moves for the next year until my seventh birthday when my father enrolled me in Tae Kwon Do classes. I achieved black belts in Han Moo Kwon Tae Kwon Do and Hakko Ryu Ju Jitsu under my venerable teacher Master Jeffrey Noel Reeder.

At the age of fourteen I began studying internal martial arts. My teachers were Rick Krause and Peter Shumway, who were the pupils of the truly exceptional Wei Lun Huang from Guangzhou, China. Shifu Huang teaches out of Orlando, Florida.

When I was studying Asian culture and languages at the The Evergreen State College in Olympia, Washington, I went on two trips to study abroad in Beijing, China. I studied with Wang Laoshi both times. Wang Laoshi, a seventy year old man who had been practicing internal martial arts day in and day out for more than thirty years, would ride his bicycle all over Beijing teaching Tai Chi, Qi Gong, and more from 4 or 5 o'clock in the morning until the afternoon each day.

I moved to Taiwan after college to teach English as a second language, and began studying with Lian Laoshi, who is a Tai Chi world champion and coach. I have also studied with Mr. Lin. Mr. Lin was a coach for the national Shui Jiao (Chinese Wrestling) team in Taiwan, and has written a comprehensive book about Shui Jiao. Unfortunately the book is written in Traditional Chinese only as of right now.

All of my instructors were exceptional.

I have personally won two World Cup Championships for Tai Chi, and competed in the 2009 World Games in Kaohsiung, Taiwan. I was a Tae Kwon Do state champion for 4 years in high school, and I went to the Tae Kwon Do National Championships hosted by the Olympic Tae Kwon Do Federation known as the United States Tae Kwon Do Union or U.S.T.U. 3 times. I failed to make the Olympic team, but I made it as far as fifth place the last year that I competed.

## A Word On Development

I have been teaching Kindergarten for three years now, and have developed a very good program for teaching a short martial arts class during my regular class schedule. I have taken a little bit of the martial arts styles (Tae Kwon Do, Tai Ji Quan, Ju Jitsu, Wu Shu, Yoga etc.) I know and have practiced for many years, and developed a 20-30minute class that children seem to both accept and enjoy. I have found that if you are too simple they won't like it, but too complicated just goes over their heads and they won't accept it.

There are elements of cardio, stretching, striking, blocking, falling, breathing techniques, ethics and more. I teach them in a way that some parts will incorporate well with others. For instance, there are many questions and answers about the falling, rolling and slightly more complicated instruction. This way I can be certain as a teacher that the students understand and will not hurt themselves. It is incorporated into the stretching routine, and it helps them learn a very helpful skill that can prevent injuries as they grow, and well into the future.

Incorporating the stretching and striking is also necessary to save time, and make a cohesive class. Learning to kick properly is much easier if you begin by showing the children (or anyone for that matter), from a seated position, the proper way to flex your toes or point them. After you show them how to flex or point in a seated position, it is a good idea to demonstrate a proper front kick, and roundhouse kick. This way they understand the connection between the seated position and the proper way to kick.

This program is not a replacement for studying at an actual martial arts school, but an introduction to some skills you would learn in such a place. The main reason for developing this introductory course is to help build interest in martial arts, and to promote safety in schools from a young age. Although it was developed to be implemented in schools, the principles learned here can be used by parents, teachers or other interested parties as well.

Classes can be integrated one, two or three times a week effectively. The kids could do a class each day, but it would be unnecessary and the repetition would be boring for them after a time. Three times a week might be a little much unless you have the time in your regular class program, and wish to incorporate the advanced techniques with more frequency.

Safety is the main concern for this class. If you do not feel that you can adequately convey the material to young students in a safe way, then do not attempt to teach it without outside guidance from someone who knows and understands the material and its application very well.

All in all, this program has been very successful at my kindergarten, and the kids really love it. After making sure that everything is safe for them and that they are working well with their classmates, it is an easy and fun tension reliever and exercise for both the kids and for you as their teacher.

## Preface

Each class runs about twenty-five minutes, and leaves around five minutes for a class discussion at the end or a game. I often play four corners, AKA go, go, go, at the end of a class with my students as an ethical conversation is not always necessary. When ethics does need to be discussed is on the first day of the first class, at the beginning of the class. It should be repeated several times until you can be certain that the students are well aware of rules and the way in which to keep a good attitude outside of class.

The ethical discussion usually consists of me asking a few simple questions, and repeating their answers with a final statement after all the questions have been asked and answered. The questions are as follows:

1.) Should you get off the white line?

2.) Should you touch your neighbor?

3.) Should you hit your classmates?

4.) Should you hit your teachers?

5.) Should you hit strangers?

6.) If you have a problem, who should you tell?

Answers and final statements should be repeated after the original questioning. The oath and final statements are as follows:

1.) Stay on the white line.

2.) Keep your hands to yourself.

3.) Don't hit your classmates.

4.) Don't hit your teachers.

5.) Don't hit strangers.

6.) If you have a problem, tell a teacher, tell your parents, tell a police officer, or tell a soldier (tell a fire fighter, the kids like to say this too).

7.) Be nice to others, and they will be nice to you.

The floor should be somewhat like the u-shape of a trapezoid. You can accomplish this by putting down some colored tape in the classroom (my tape is white) where you wish to practice. Here is an example of the layout:

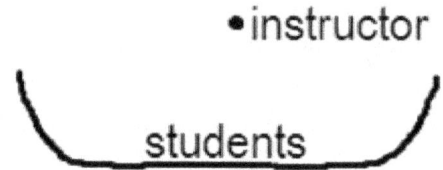

There may be a need for more space for the students in which case you can make a second row behind the main line. It would look like this:

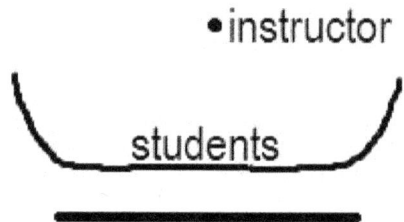

The students should have about an arms width of room to maneuver. This will help them keep enough distance to avoid hitting or bumping into each other during class.

Always be sure that the students stay on the line, and are a good distance from their neighbor. They tend to wander, which can lead to accidents. It is best to give some strict rules for dealing with the students in this capacity. If a student leaves the taped floor, I generally tell them to get back on it. If it happens more than once, I make them go sit down. The same goes for touching other students. After some time I will invite them to come back to the class, so long as they understand that they need to stay in their place.

It would be a good idea to make some sharpie "X"s on the colored tape. This way the students will know exactly where they need to be. I don't use them in my class, but the students are very well behaved. With a less disciplined class it might be necessary at the beginning, but over time they might not be needed.

All material is covered in pictures as well, with commands. The commands must be said and repeated by the children to help complete the circle of visual, auditory and kinesthetic learning. It is also important to follow the sequence as outlined in the text. Everything has been carefully reviewed to make sure that the class is a very cohesive learning experience.

# Units 1 & 2: Starting, Stretching and the Warm-up, and Supplementary Intermissions

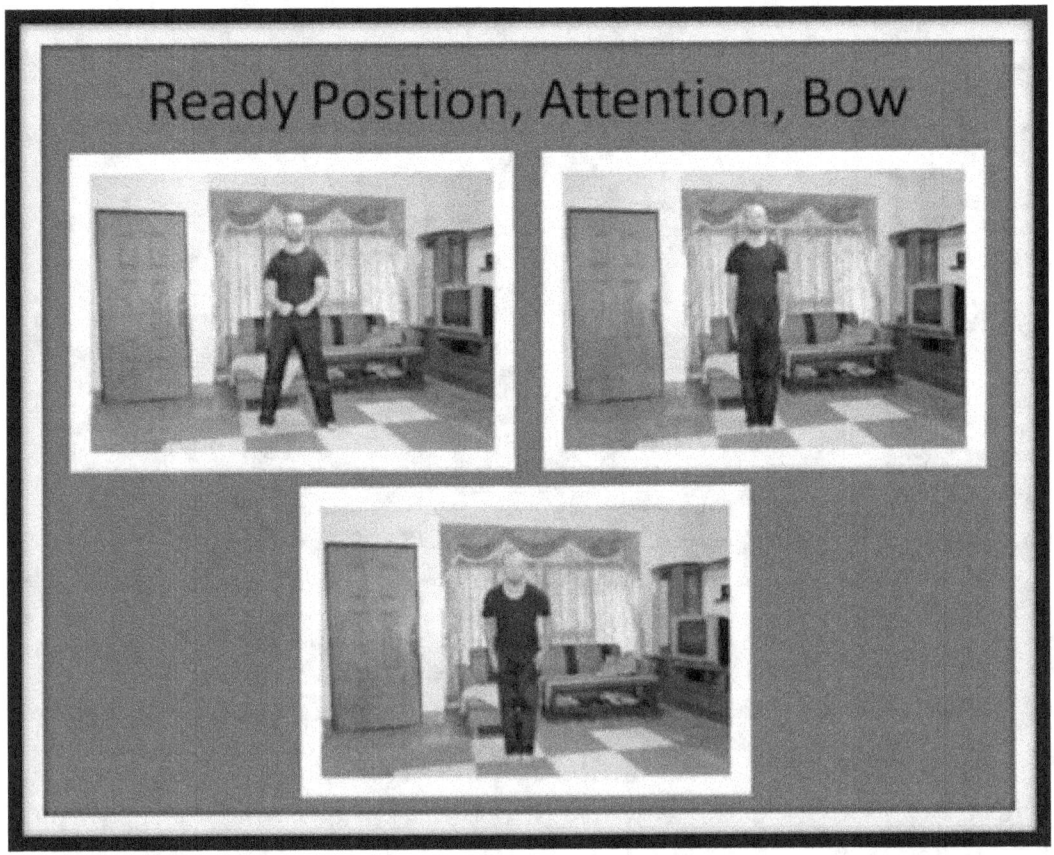

Ready Position, Attention, Bow

Begin and end each class with a formal bow in and out to help establish the class. An easy warm-up to begin with is jumping jacks. Running in place is also a good way to start the class, or maybe running a few small laps around the room. Once you have done about thirty to fifty seconds of running in place, jogged around the room two or three times or twenty-five jumping jacks, warming up the joints is important. Start by moving your head forward and back, and then side to side. Have the children repeat the instructions as you say them. This is a good way for them to learn and imbed what they are learning.

Notes

# Jumping Jacks

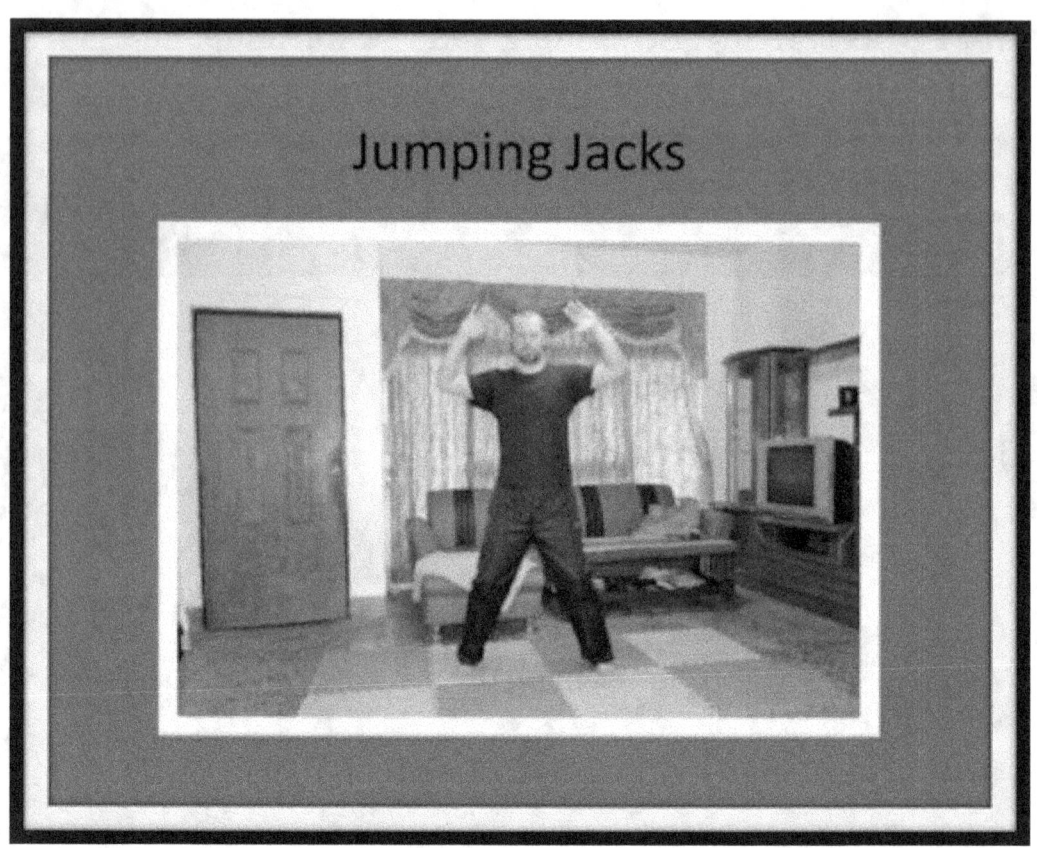

Continue warming up the joints by making circles at the neck, wrists, elbows, shoulders, waist and back, knees and then finally the ankles. For the ankles, first touch the toe and then the heel to the ground as if you were practicing ballet. The front toe goes down, and then the heel goes down as you lift the toe. Then squish a bug. Take the front toe and twist your ankle back and forth as though you were squishing a cockroach. Repeat the same motion with the heel down.

Notes

_____

_____

_____

_____

_____

_____

# Roll your wrists, elbows, shoulders, and neck

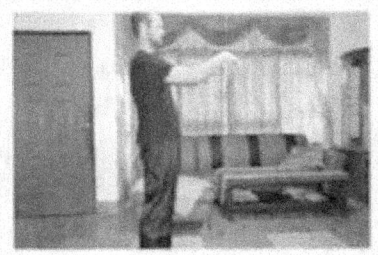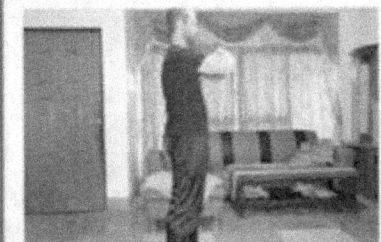

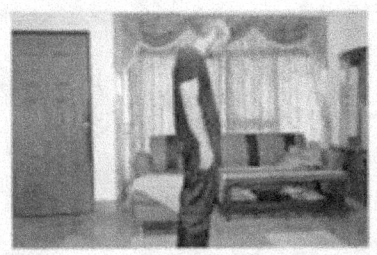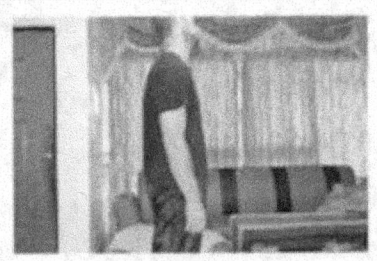

# Roll your body at the waist, then hips

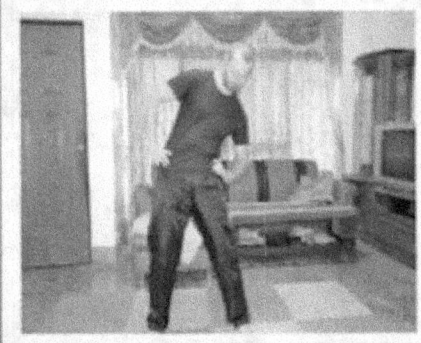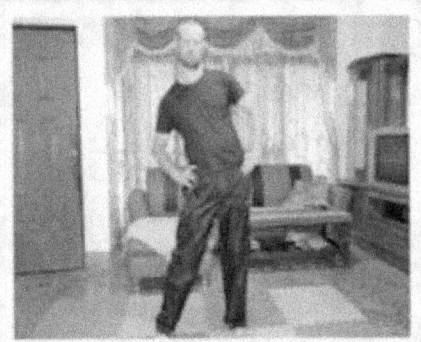

# Bend your knees, and make circles

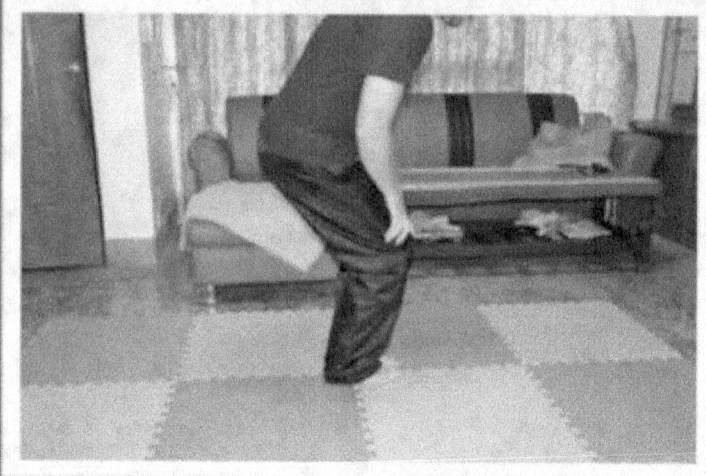

Bend and straighten a few times, and make circles

# Squash a bug with your toe
# Squash a bug with your heel

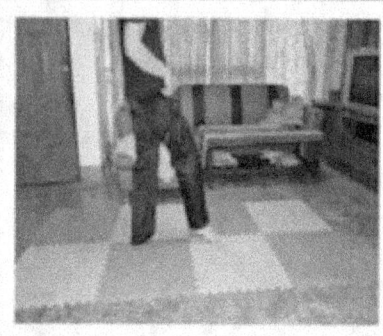 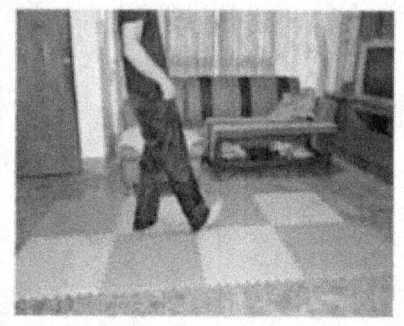

Switch between toe and heel a few times first

After the warm-up it's time to stretch. Along with everything in class, nothing should be forced, especially stretching. Make sure both the kids and you only do what is comfortable. Never try to push them too far, and don't try to overdo anything yourself. Over time they will improve naturally, as will you.

Begin by lifting your hands up with fingers pointed toward the ceiling and stand up on your toes. Then slowly come back down, let the hands fall first in front and finally down to your feet. Slowly come back up and relax. Now, split your feet apart about three feet (probably a foot for the little ones), and put your hands down in the middle. Then lean to each side and hold your leg.

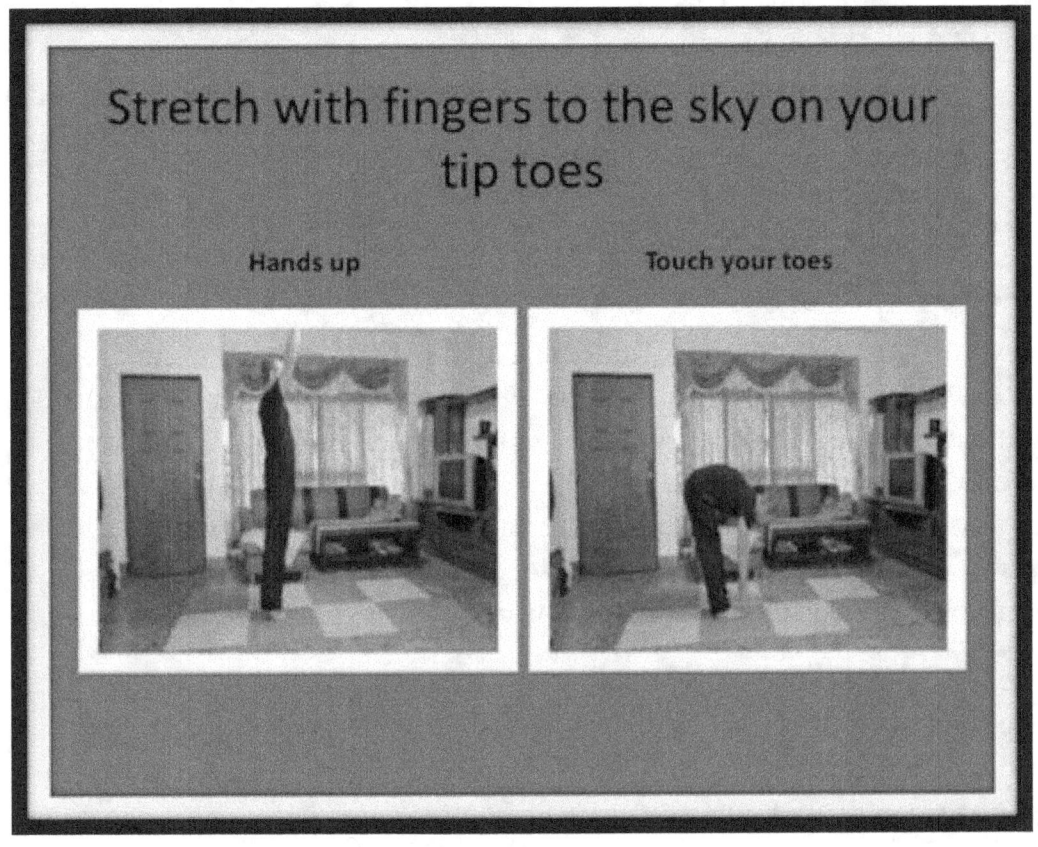

Notes

_____

_____

_____

_____

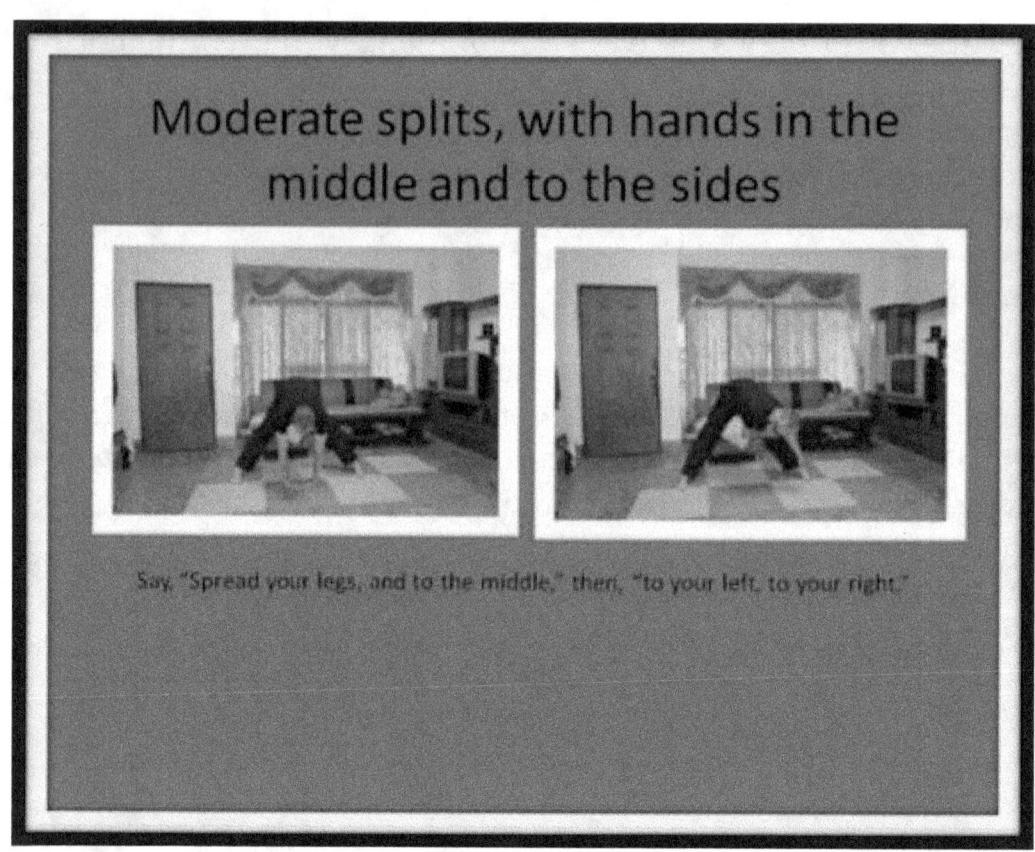

**Moderate splits, with hands in the middle and to the sides**

Say, "Spread your legs, and to the middle," then, "to your left, to your right."

Now you can begin spreading the eagles wings and hugging a tree. Go down to one side in a crouch. The toe of the other leg should be pointing straight up. Spread your arms with one close to your straight leg, and the other extended beyond your bent leg. Come forward as you begin to bend the straight leg and move your torso slowly up. Now your arms should be over your knee in a hug position, as though you are holding a ball or hugging a tree.

These techniques can be done in a few different ways, but with the younger students (age 3-4) just work on getting them to crouch on one side and lunge on the other. It will be hard enough for them to get into the proper position at the beginning.

Notes

_____

_____

_____

_____

# Down and to the side

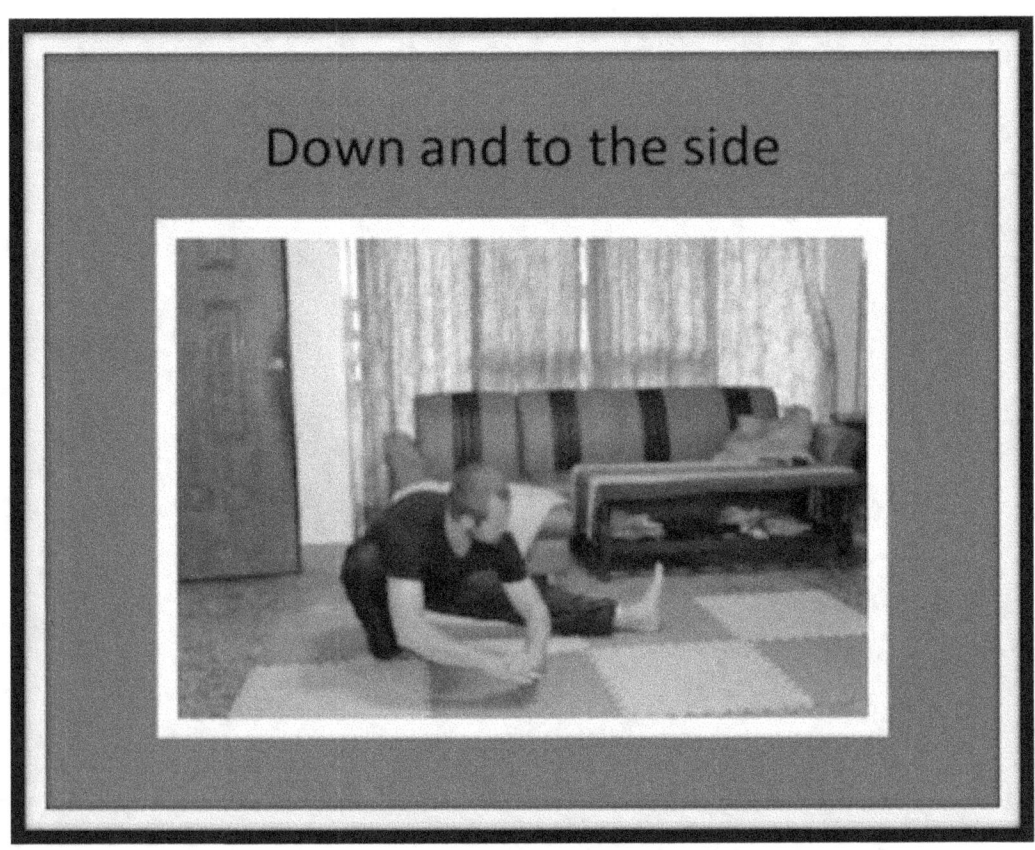

Notes

# Up and to the other side

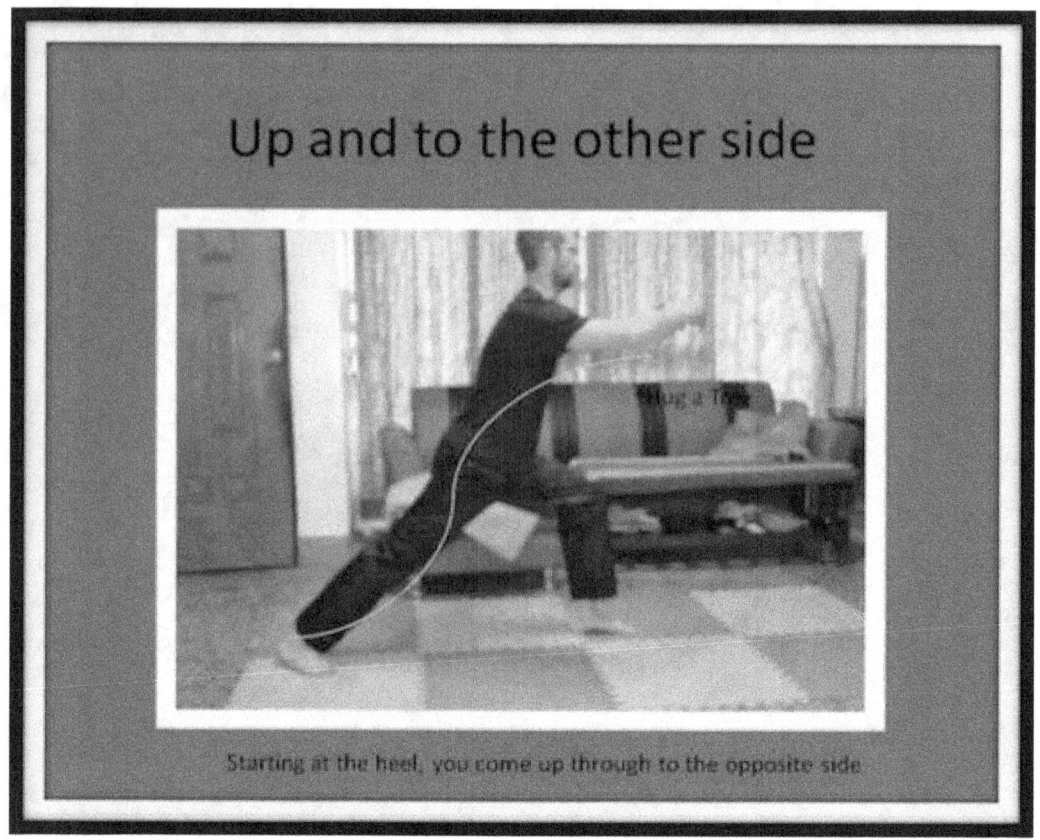

Starting at the heel, you come up through to the opposite side

After finishing hugging the tree and spreading the eagle's wings, put your hands back in between your legs and feet and spread your legs as far as you can. Sit down in a split and stretch to the middle and sides. Bring your feet together after stretching for a minute or two, into a butterfly position. Tell the children to, "flap their butterfly wings."

The legs move up and down at the knees when you flap your butterfly wings. After some good flapping, put your head down in the middle and side to side. Next, you can extend the legs to a diamond shape and stretch to the middle and sides.

Stretch in diamond shape for a minute or two, and then extend both legs forward and reach to touch your ankles. If that is easy for the kids, tell them to touch their toes. If that is easy, tell them to touch the balls of their feet (most of the kindergarteners cannot touch the balls of their feet, let alone their toes).

If you are teaching an older class of kids, you can proceed to stretching one leg at a time. Extend one leg with your other leg tucked into the side of the extended leg and touch your toes. Once you have adequately stretched the hamstrings, cross one leg over the other and twist your back.

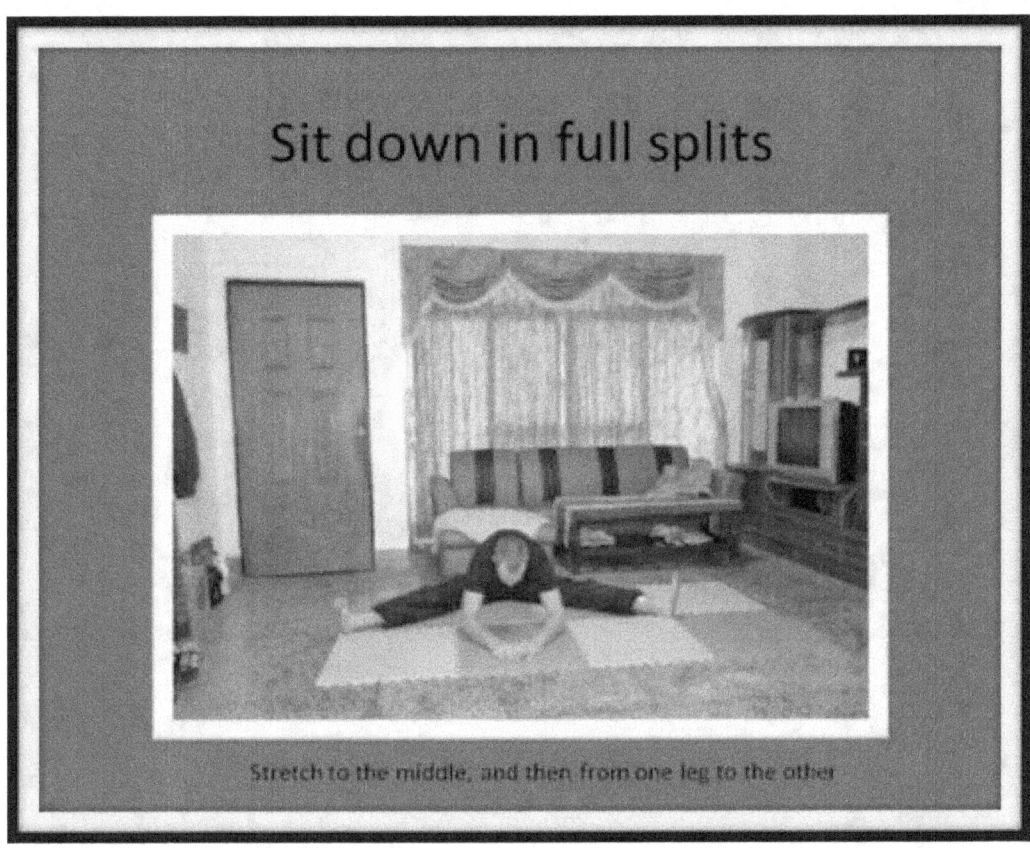

Sit down in full splits

Stretch to the middle, and then from one leg to the other

Notes

_____

_____

_____

_____

_____

_____

_____

_____

_____

_____

_____

_____

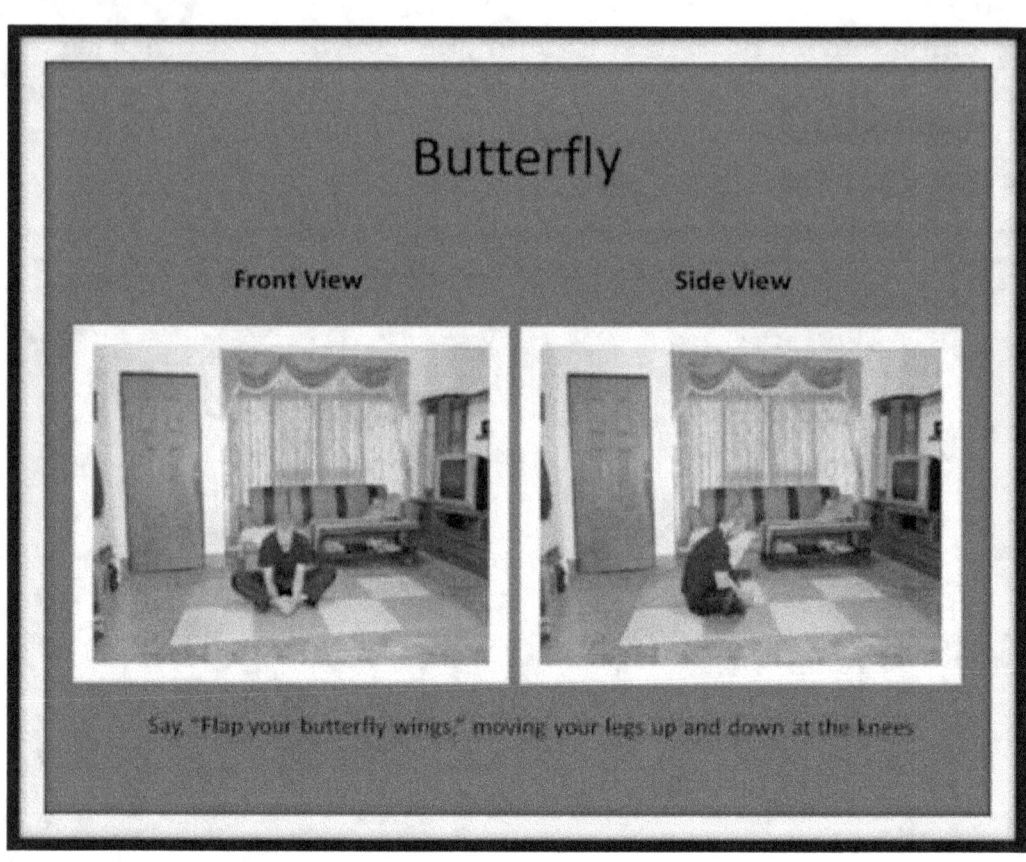

## Butterfly

**Front View**

**Side View**

Say, "Flap your butterfly wings," moving your legs up and down at the knees

Notes

_____

_____

_____

_____

_____

_____

_____

_____

_____

_____

_____

_____

_____

_____

_____

_____

_____

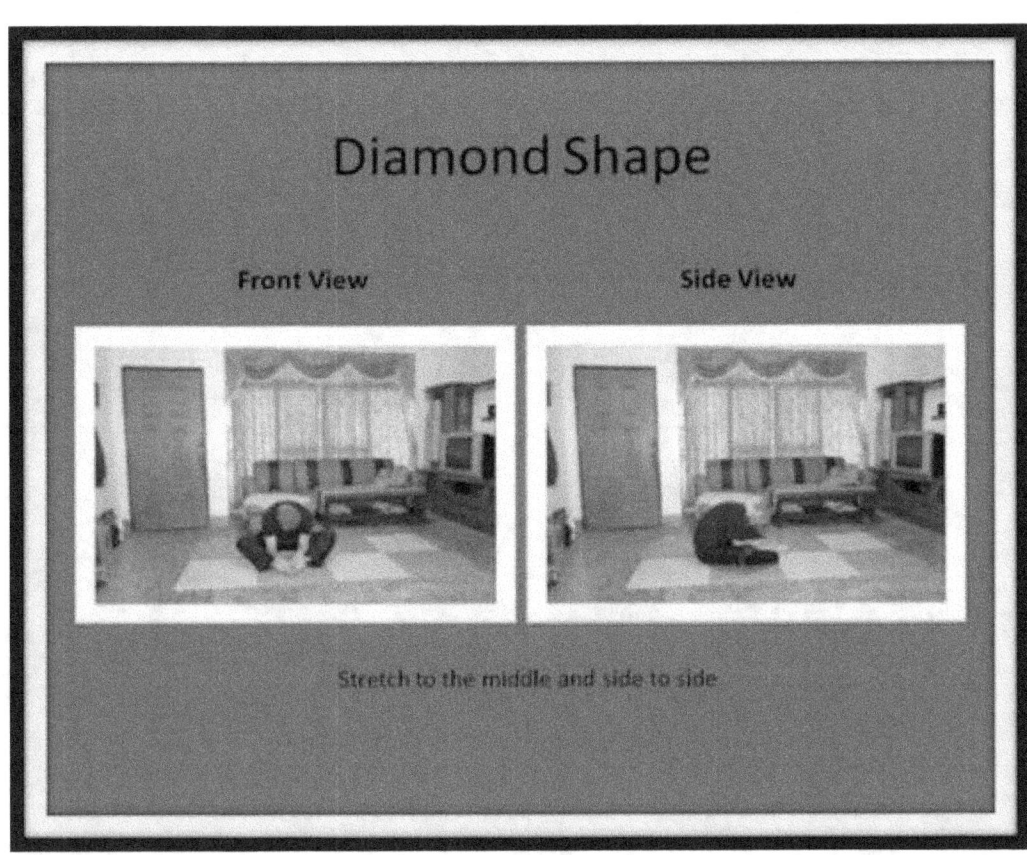

Notes

_____

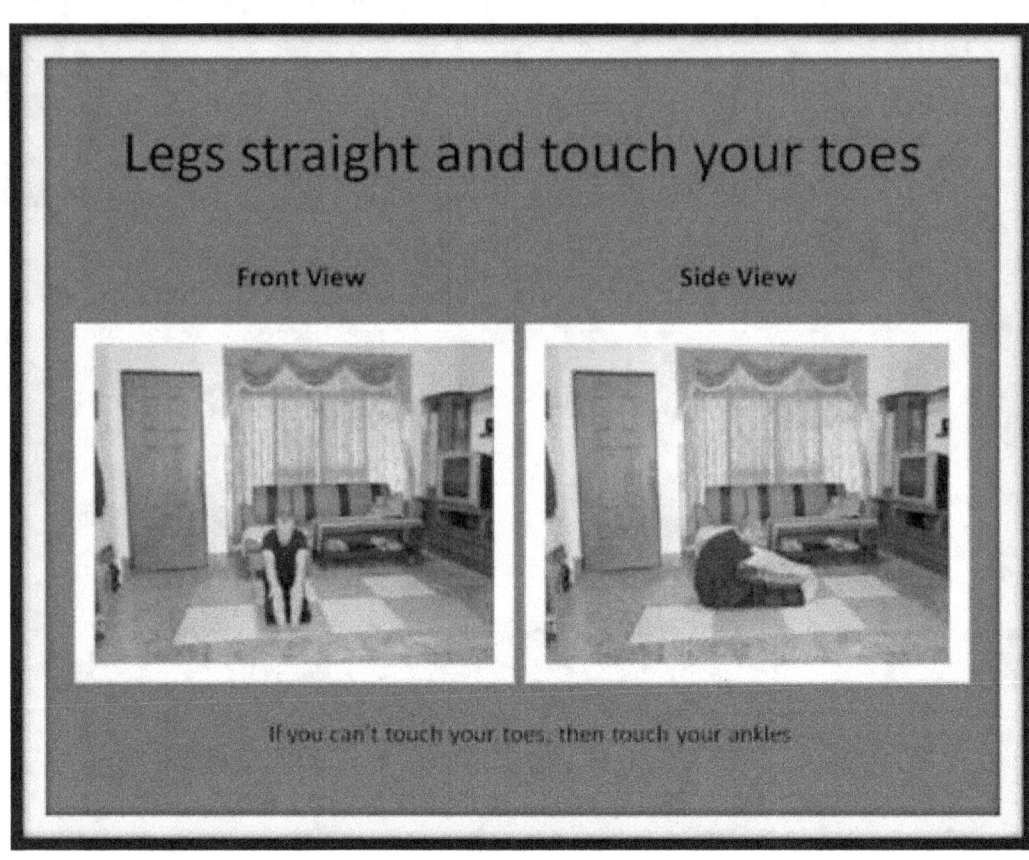

Notes

_____
_____
_____
_____
_____
_____
_____
_____
_____
_____
_____
_____
_____
_____
_____
_____
_____
_____

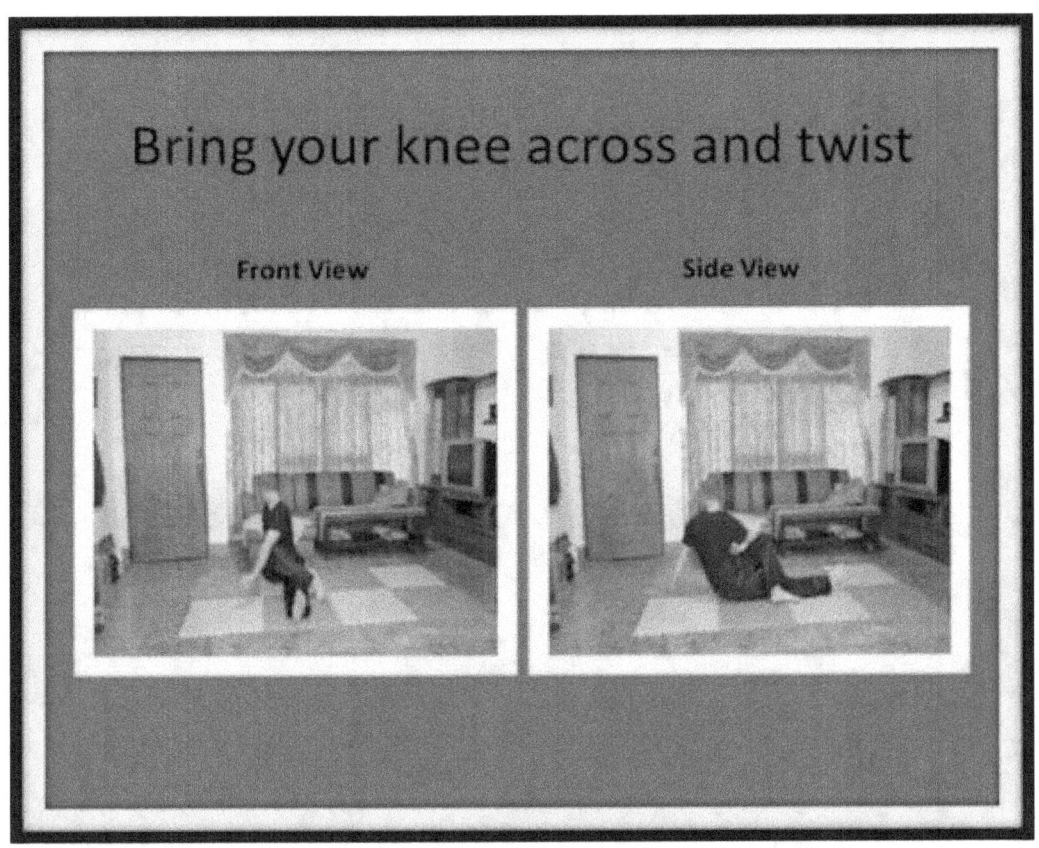

Bring your knee across and twist

Front View       Side View

Now it's time to lie down. When you lie down, put your hands above your head and stretch from your toes through to your fingertips. Then bring one knee up into your chest, followed by the other and finally both knees. For older classes, have the students bring their feet over and above their head in what is sometimes referred to as the woodcutting position or the plough in yoga.

Finish the lying with the back down segment of stretching, and you can lean to one side with one leg tucked under and the other being gripped at the heel by the hand on the same side with the same leg. Extend your leg as far as you can, and tell the kids to do the same. Next, put your hand around the leg and foot and pull it down towards your chest. I used to tell my students at this point to kiss their toes to be funny, but that is not a good idea. The kids love it, and you will see many toe suckers if you do this.

Bring your knees to your chest

One at a time

Both knees

Bring your head toward your knee

Notes

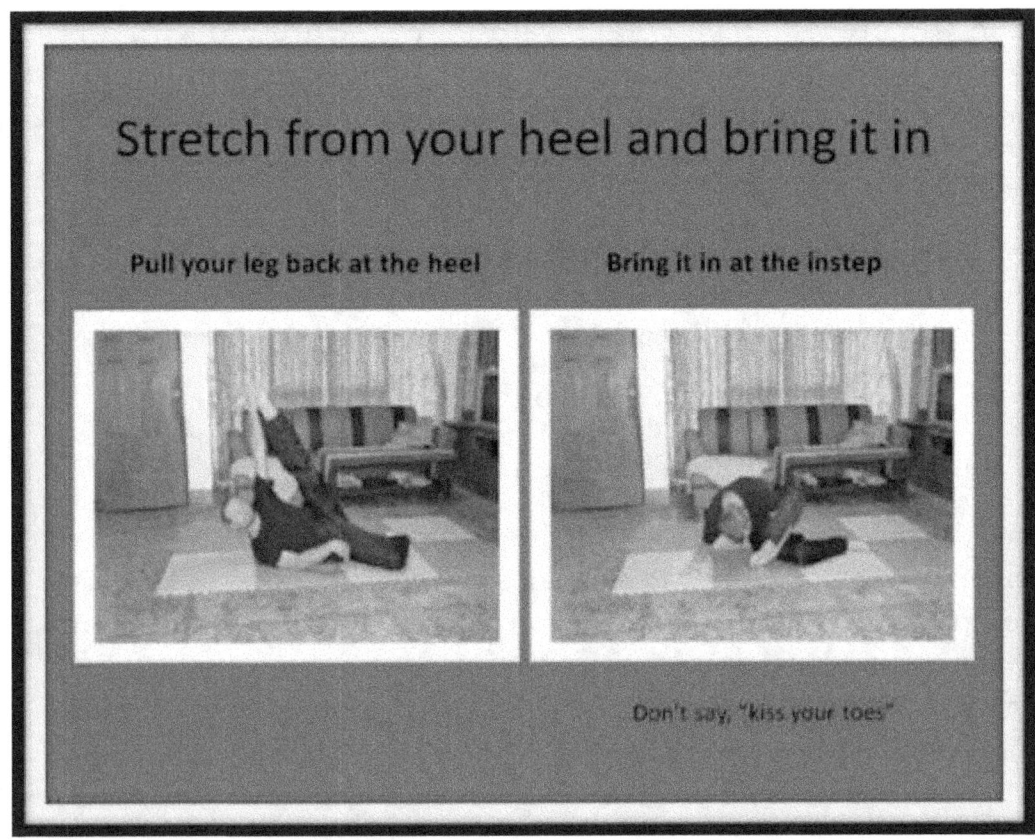

Stretch from your heel and bring it in

Pull your leg back at the heel

Bring it in at the instep

Don't say, "kiss your toes"

After extending and retracting the legs on each side it's time to learn back falls and side falls.

*+Falling; intermission #1 between stretching routine* **Unit 2**

Falling is a very important activity for the kids. If they learn and practice how to fall properly, it will help them avoid many accidents. I have seen the effectiveness of teaching the kids how to fall, and how much they avoid injuries on the playground as a result.

First, sit in a half lotus position with one leg folded over the other. This position will help maintain balance when falling backwards, or to the side. Next, you cross your arms in front of your chest making an "X". Tuck your chin into your neck and fall back. Slap the ground with your palms face down.  Your arms should be no more than forty-five degrees away from your body. You can practice first by hitting the ground with your hands at your sides while sitting down.

When you are falling you don't want to hit the ground with any part of your body other than your back or side and your palm. Reinforce this idea with the kids by asking these questions;

1.) Do you hit the ground with your head? No

2.) Do you hit the ground with your elbow? No

3.) Do you hit the ground with your chest? No

4.) Do you hit the ground with your hands? Yes

5.) Do you hit the ground with your back? Yes

As with the questions about hitting others and if you have a problem, you don't have to ask these questions every class. You should ask them for at least 5 or 6 classes at the beginning, and remember to ask them every so often as a reminder. It will help both them and yourself sink in the idea of protecting your more vulnerable areas when falling.

Side falls are similar to back falls, but you only bring one hand up and across your chest. Look at the palm of your hand and put your head down with your chin in your neck. Fall to the same side as the hand you are holding up and strike the ground with the palm of your hand.

Notes

_____

_____

_____

_____

_____

_____

_____

_____

_____

_____

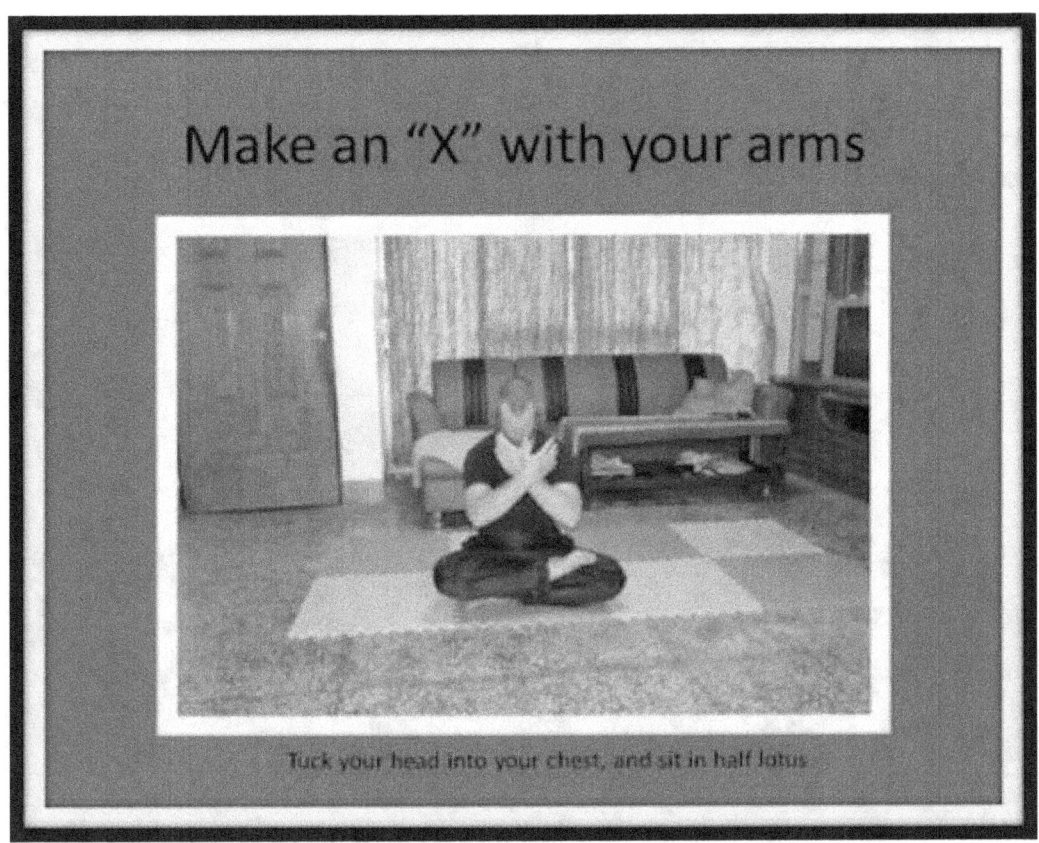

Make an "X" with your arms

Tuck your head into your chest, and sit in half lotus

Notes

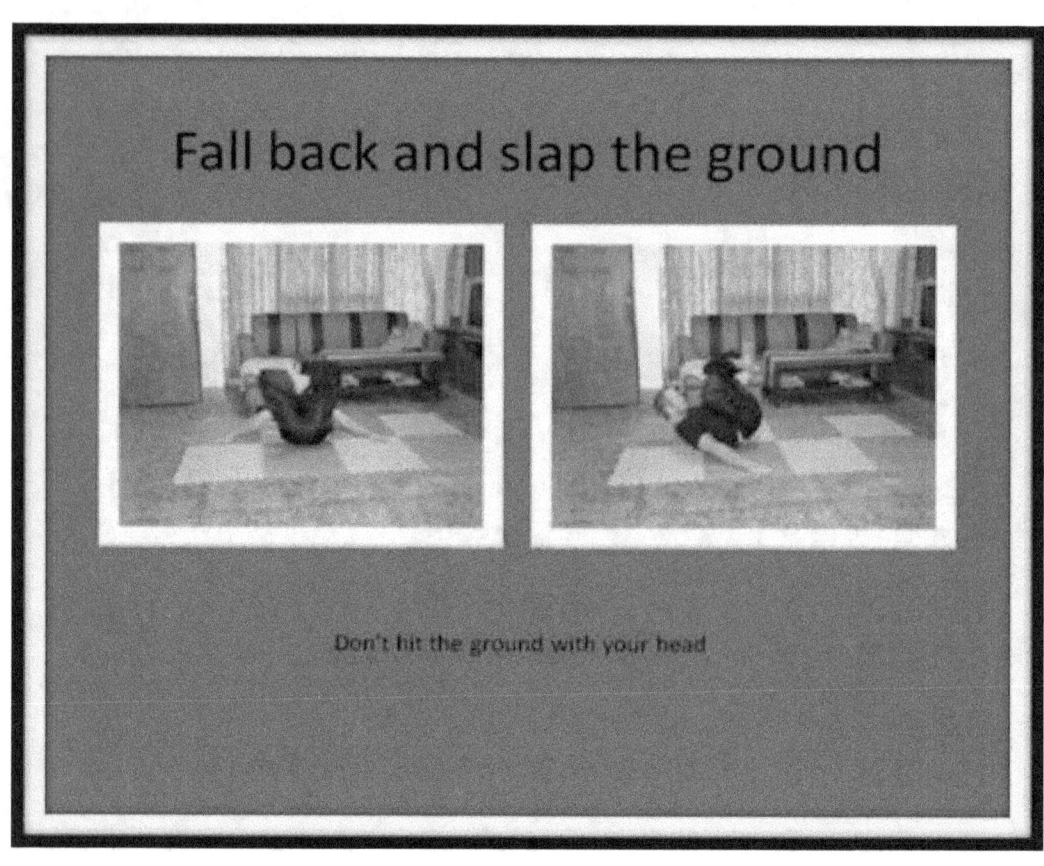

Fall back and slap the ground

Don't hit the ground with your head

Notes

_____
_____
_____
_____
_____
_____
_____
_____
_____
_____
_____
_____
_____
_____
_____
_____
_____

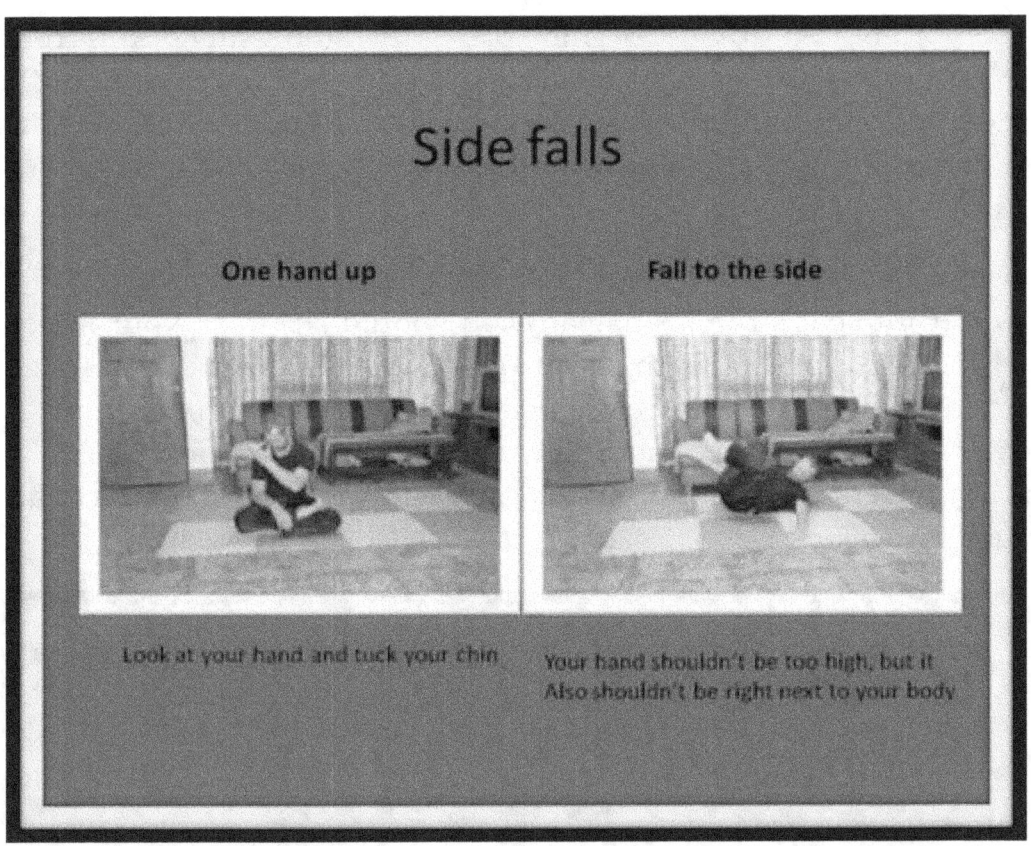

Front falls are covered in the supplementary material **Unit 6**.

The children really like this section, and it is the most important for their safety. When I was a child I broke my jaw in kindergarten while running through the halls. Even though you may try your best to keep children from running, chances are they will at some point be running. Learning to fall teaches them how to put their hands out in a safe way, and will help them protect themselves from injury.

After practicing falls, it's time to turn on to your belly and go through cobra, lion, cat, frog and dog stretches. Cobra stretches the lower back. You begin by lying flat on your stomach, and then raising your torso onto your elbows. After staying there for a moment, go back down and place your palms flat. Come all the way up into cobra, and let the kids make hissing noises. Look to your left and right respectively, before moving into lion stretch.

In lion stretch you move directly back on to your knees with your posterior pointed up and behind you. Your hands stay out in front on the ground as you face the floor and pull your lower back in the opposite position from where you were stretching in cobra. As with the snake sounds, you can have the children roar like little lions here.

Once you've stretched in this position for some time, do not transfer into cat stretch. Instead, you should sit up on your knees with your feet placed so that your posterior is on your heels and ankles. Your toes are therefore flexed underneath. This teaches how your toes and feet should be when performing a front kick, and transversely, how you should position your feet to perform a roundhouse kick.

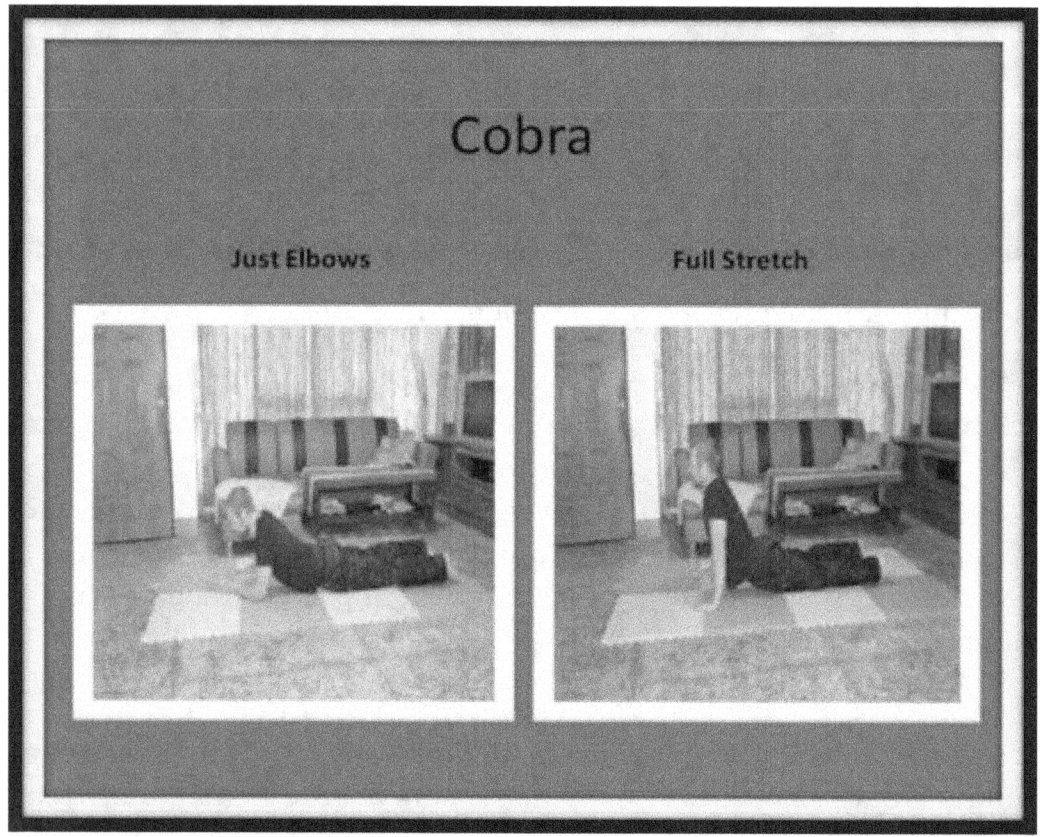

Notes

_____

_____

_____

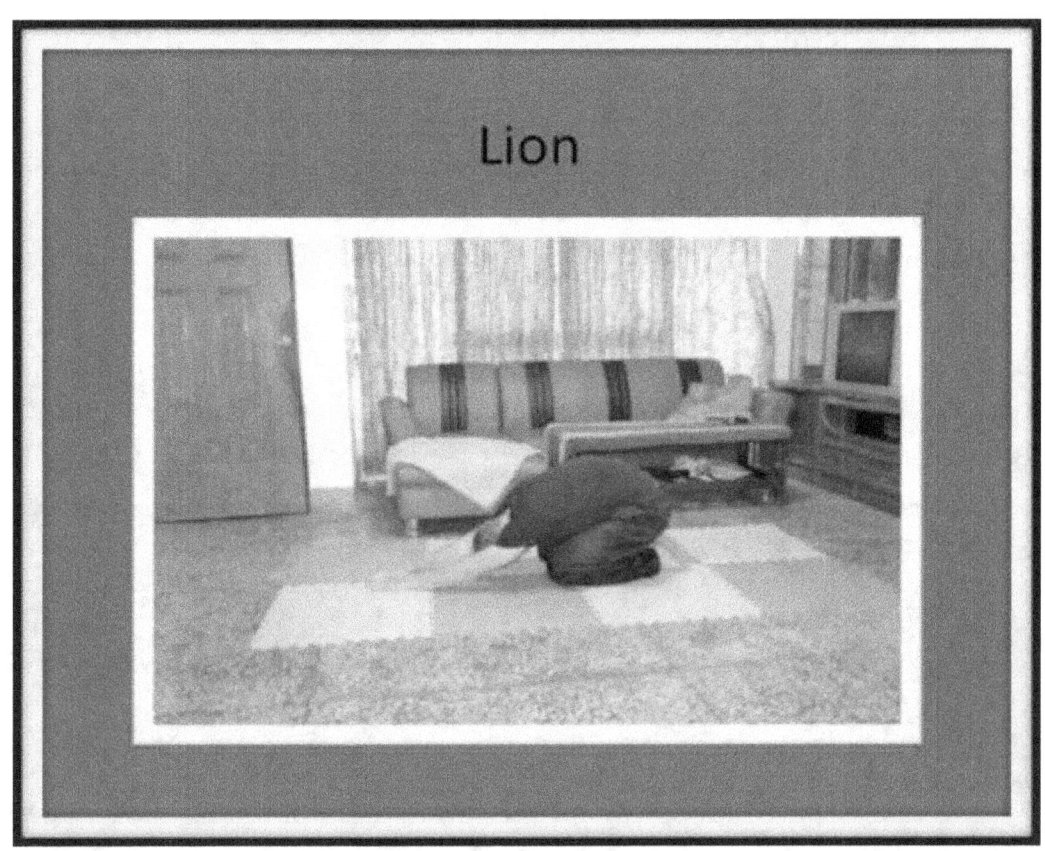

Lion

*+Hand Techniques; intermission #2 between stretching routine*

From this position you can show the children some basic wrist grip techniques. The first thing is to put your hands on your legs just above the knees. Pull the hands up first at the wrists, as though your fingertips were like the bristles of a paintbrush just floating back across your legs. Then bring both hands directly up and out. You should be holding your hands slightly bent in front of your body and shoulder high. The palms should be facing each other with fingers spread apart.

Now scratch your ear. Bring your hands, one at a time, back in a motion as though you were scratching your ear. Next perform a chop to the neck of your imaginary opponent with one hand while placing the other at your waist. At this point you can change the position of your feet so that you're sitting on the insteps of your feet. When you begin teaching the advanced material, wait to change your position until after you've finished two techniques.

The second technique begins the same as though your fingertips are a paintbrush, and then you raise your hands in front of you facing each other. This time you can bring one hand to the waist of the same side. You should bring the other hand across your chest and neck to your opposite ear, and with the hand at the ear, perform a cross chop to the neck of your invisible adversary.

All hand techniques are performed without a partner. It is fun for the kids to practice them even though they don't understand the purpose of each technique. It teaches a valuable repetition which they can apply later, if they wish to pursue a martial arts class.

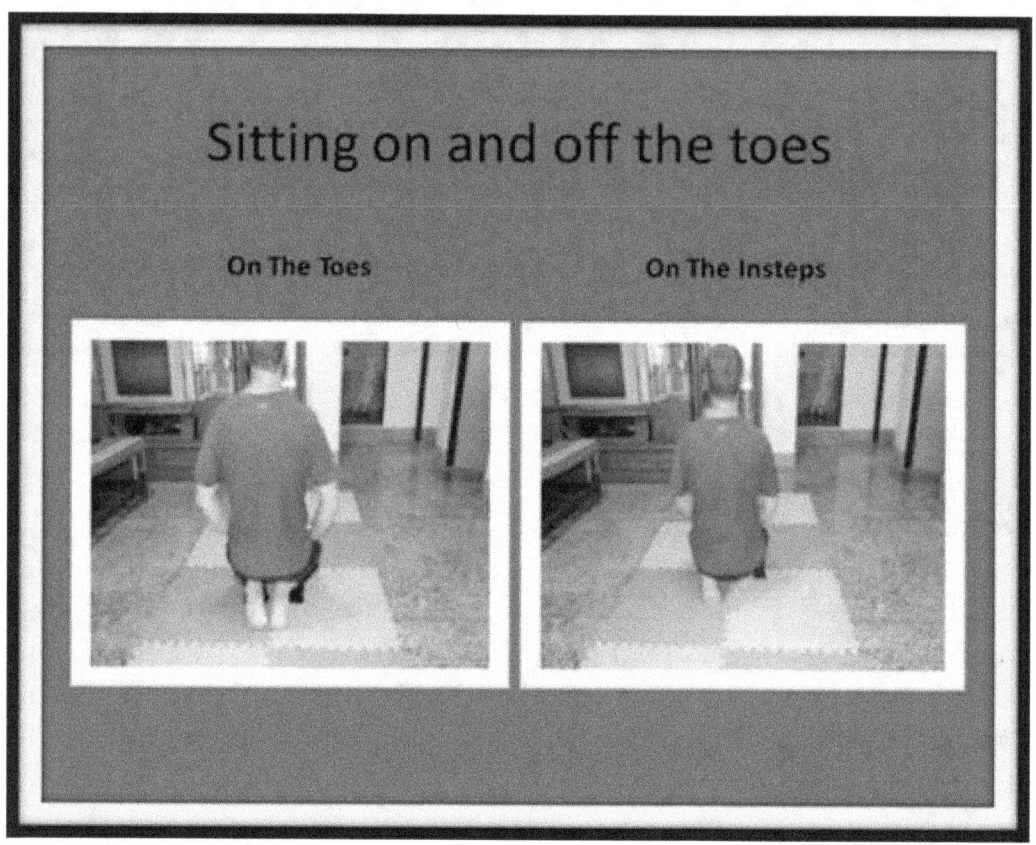

Sitting on and off the toes

On The Toes        On The Insteps

Notes

_____

_____

_____

_____

_____

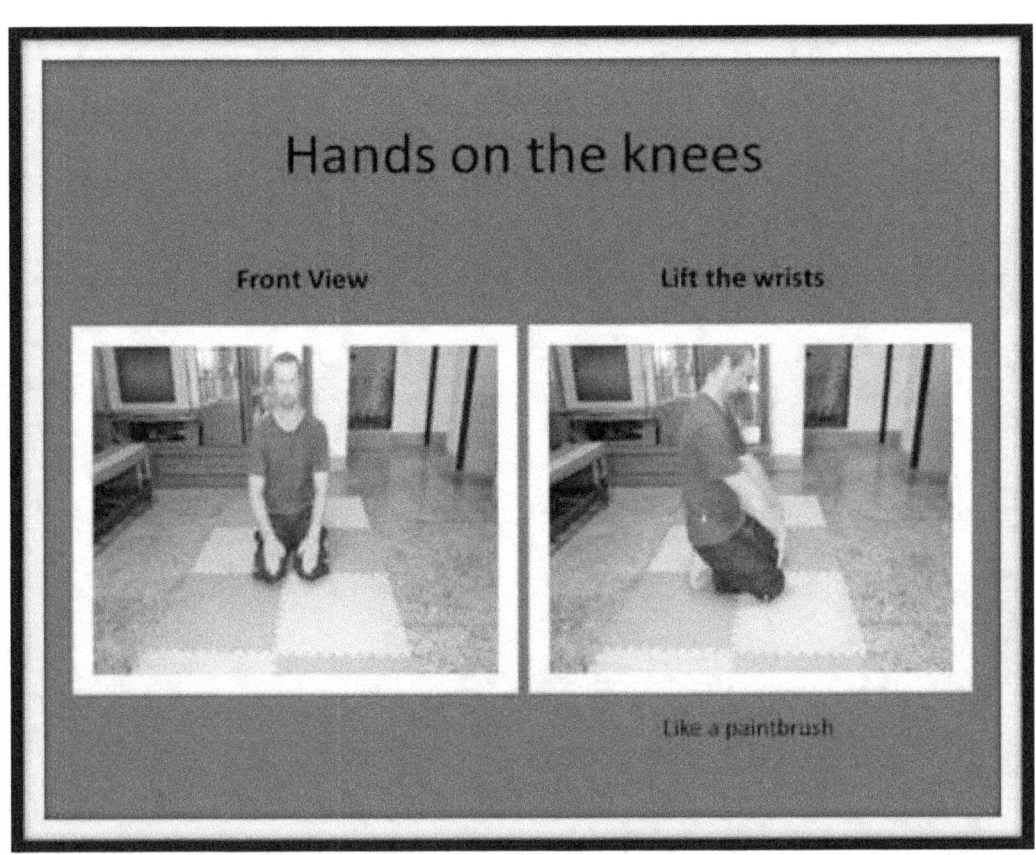

Notes

_____
_____
_____
_____
_____
_____
_____
_____
_____
_____
_____
_____
_____
_____
_____
_____

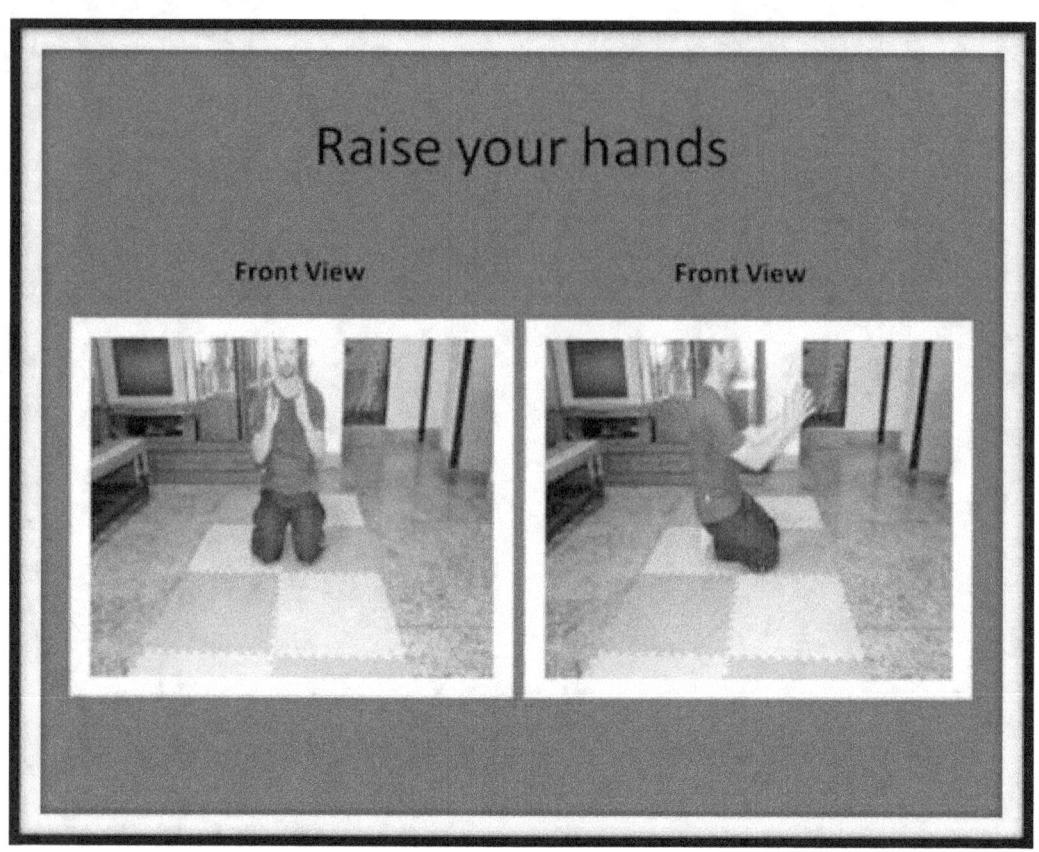

Notes

_____

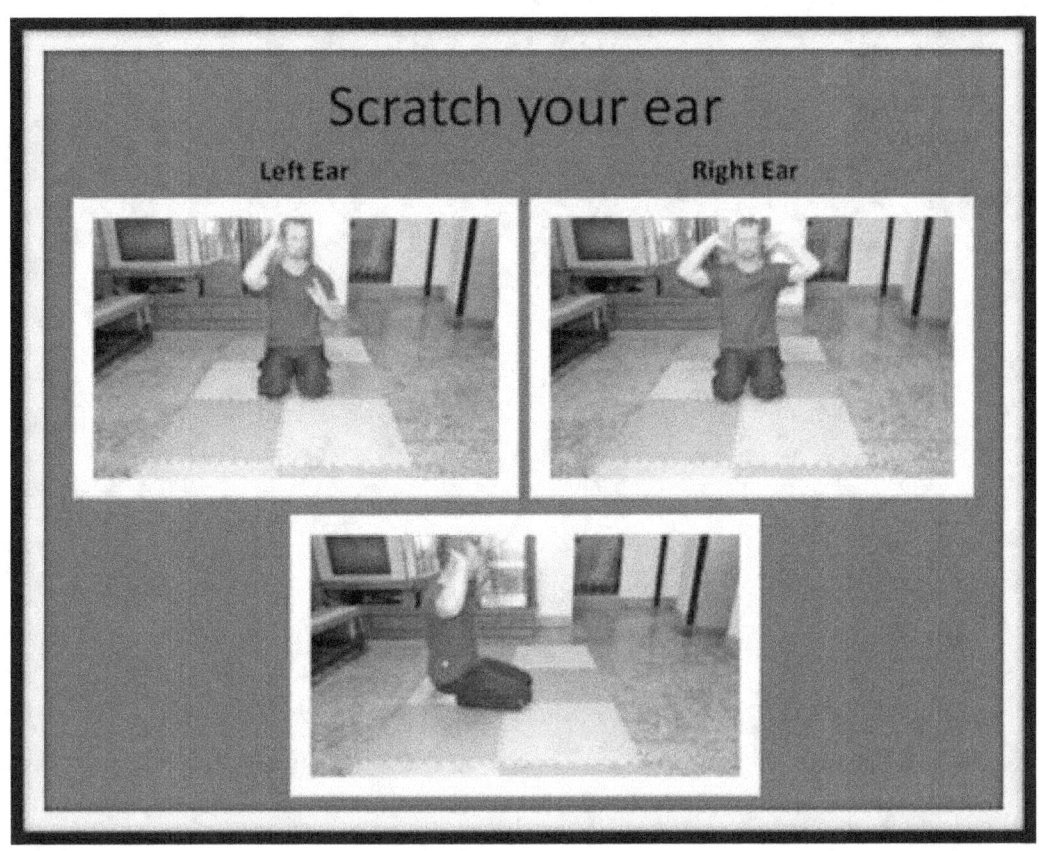

Notes

_____
_____
_____
_____
_____
_____
_____
_____
_____
_____
_____
_____
_____
_____
_____

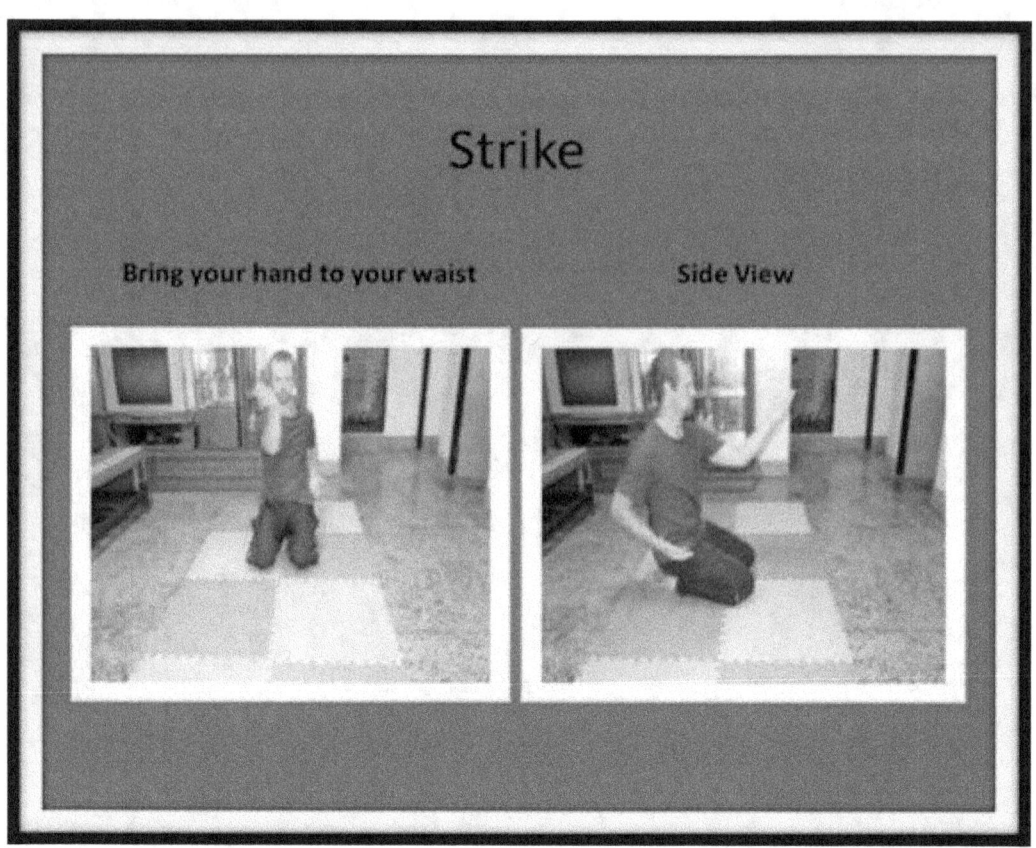

Notes

_____

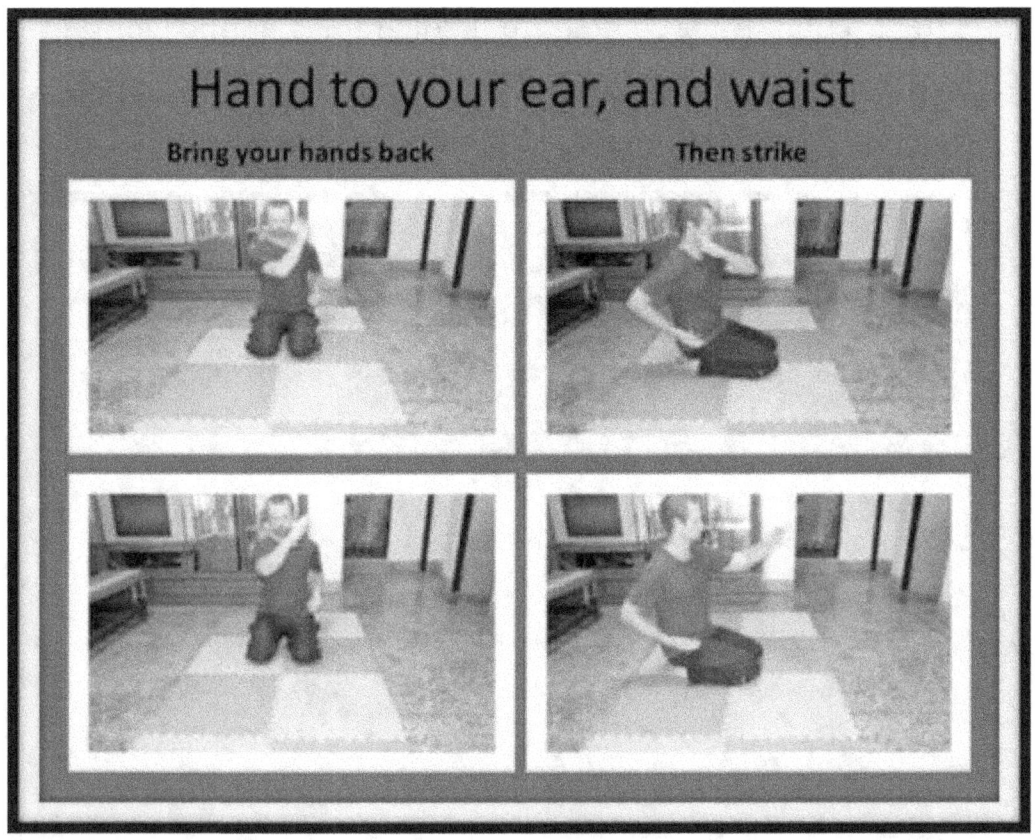

**Hand to your ear, and waist**

Bring your hands back | Then strike

From the seated position, move forward onto your hands with your posterior directly over your knees. This is cat position, and the kids enjoy meowing like cats here. Roll your shoulders in both directions, and you can scrunch your neck a bit to feel the stretch their as well.

Spread your legs apart and place your upper body weight on your elbows. This is frog position. In frog position, you are trying to stretch the hips. Hip flexibility is important for kicking and other physical activities. Especially sidekicks, which are not covered in this program, will benefit from this position.

The last position, sometimes refered to as downward dog, is the dog position. You make the shape of an arc with your body, and both your hands and feet are on the ground. In dog position you are stretching your ankles, calves and hamstrings primarily.

Slowly walk your hands back and rise from your waist up stacking each vertebra one at a time as you come up. This is the end of the stretching section. After coming up, I sometimes bounce for a little

bit to warm up again. It's good for the joints to be nice and loose as you perform the next section of class.

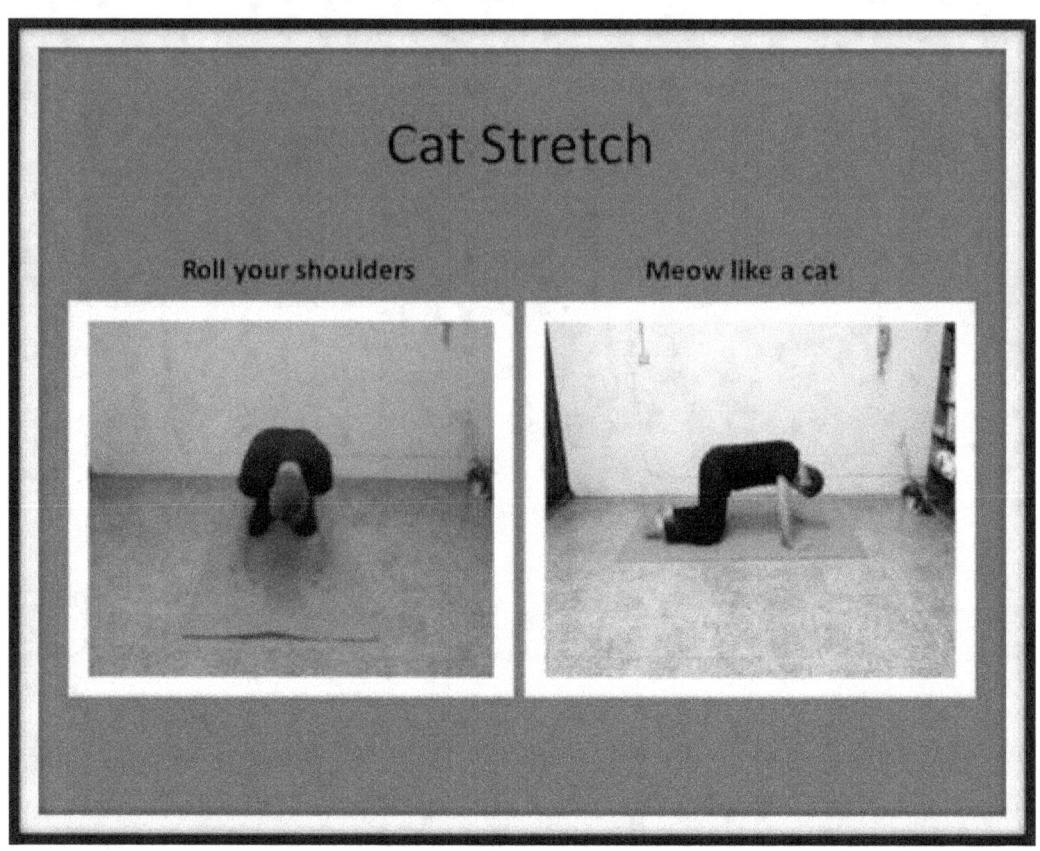

Notes

_____

_____

_____

_____

_____

_____

_____

_____

_____

_____

_____

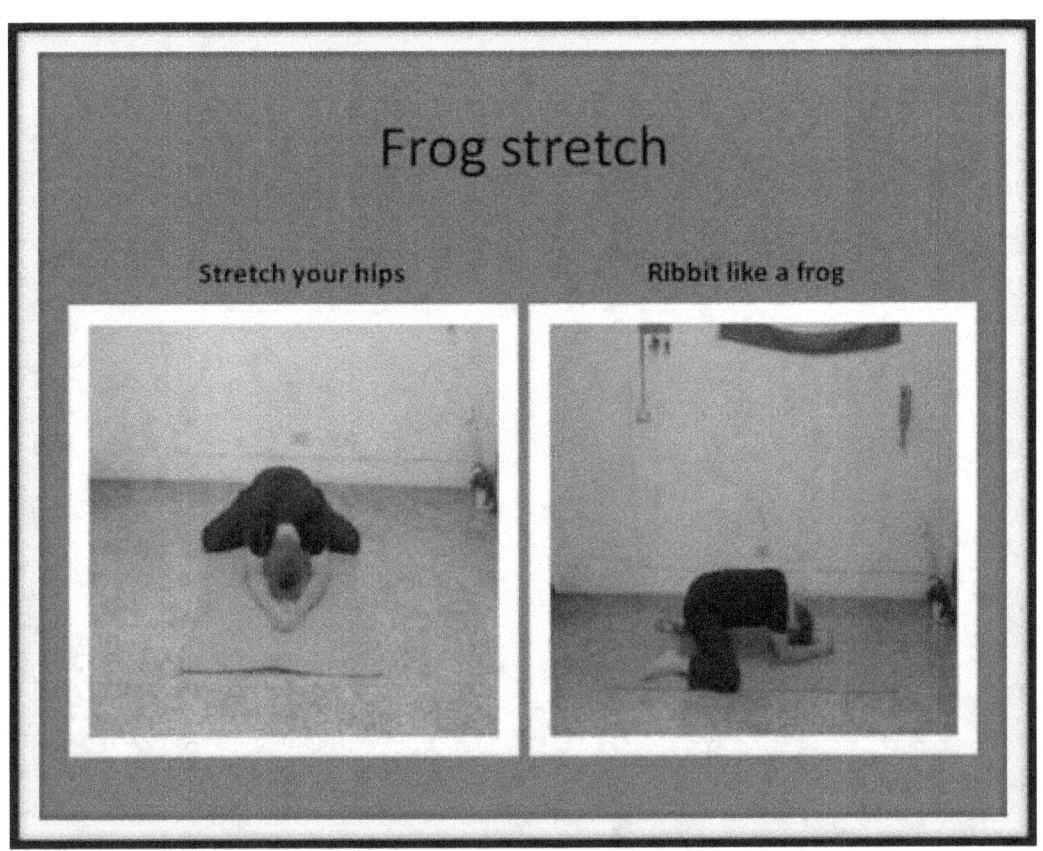

Notes

_____
_____
_____
_____
_____
_____
_____
_____
_____
_____
_____
_____
_____
_____
_____
_____

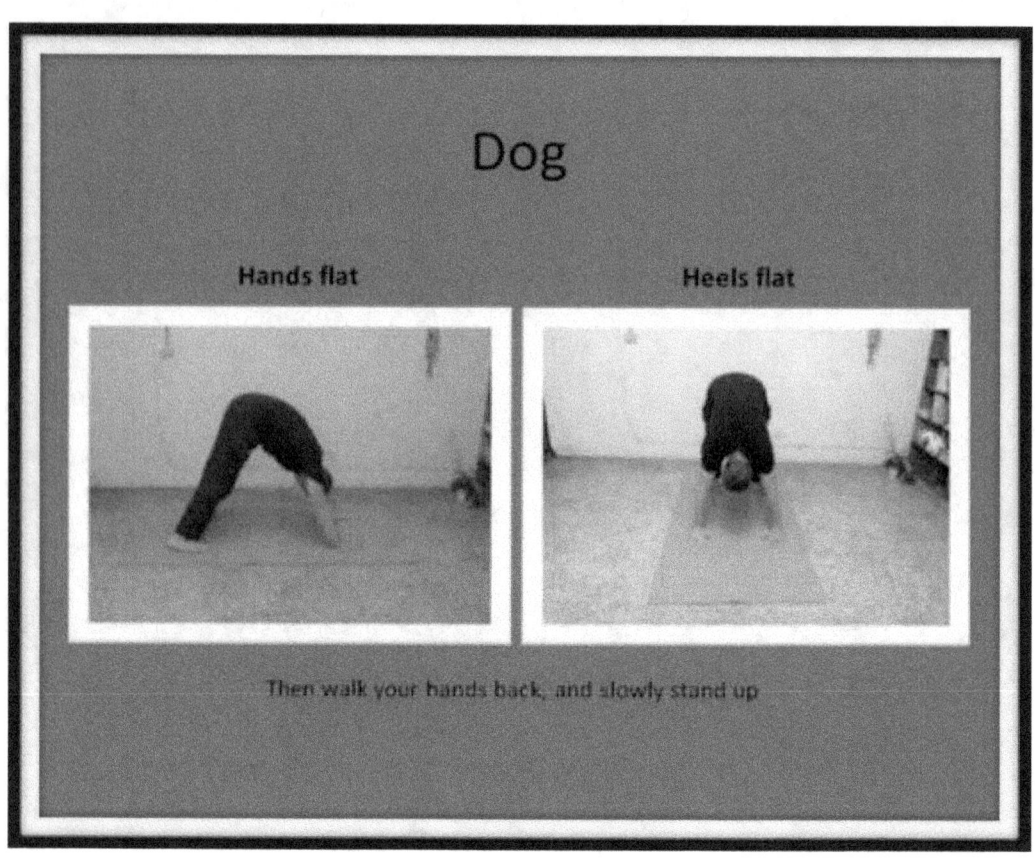

Notes

# Notes

## Unit 3: Stances

At the beginning of the class, you will introduce ready position, which is done to bring uniformity to the class. Both feet are shoulder width apart, and facing a little less than a 45° angle away from the body. Your hands should be in front of your hips with both fists clenched.

From ready position you will transition into the other stances. The first stance to practice is horse stance. Your feet are placed about two times that of shoulder width apart, and your hands go to your waist. The feet should be parallel and facing forward. It is called horse stance, because it resembles riding a horse, but it didn't actually come from riding horses. It was most likely developed by Chinese soldiers to create a strong base from which to take down a Mongolian soldier on horseback.

When transitioning between stances, go back and forth between ready position and horse stance. Then you can transition from ready position and fighting stance, and so on and so forth many times over. Getting in and out of position is good practice, and it is quite a lot of fun for the kids. Do this with each position as the class progresses.

Notes

_____

_____

_____

_____

_____

_____

_____

_____

_____

_____

_____

_____

_____

_____

From ready position again, the next stance is called fighting stance. In fighting stance you place one foot forward and the other directly behind it. The toe of the forward foot faces your adversary, while the other foot is about 90° or less in contrast to the forward foot. Fighting stance can be performed on either the right or left side, and switching between the two is encouraged, if not necessary.

In fighting stance, your hands are placed with the one over your rear foot guarding your face, and the other guarding your torso. The hands should be clenched in fists as with ready position and horse stance unless otherwise directed.

The weight should be distributed equally in both horse stance and ready stance. However, in fighting stance the weight should be around 70% on the rear leg, and 30% on the front leg. This can change depending on the movement you intend to make, but generally the rule is 70-30.

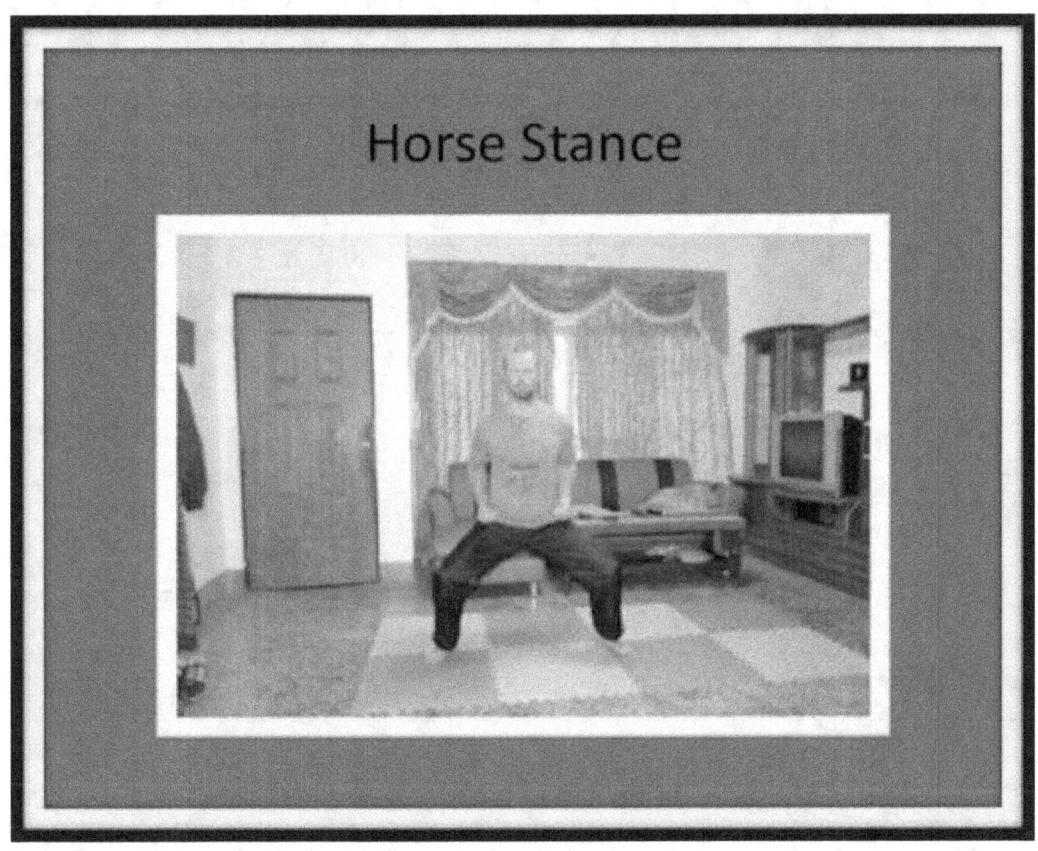

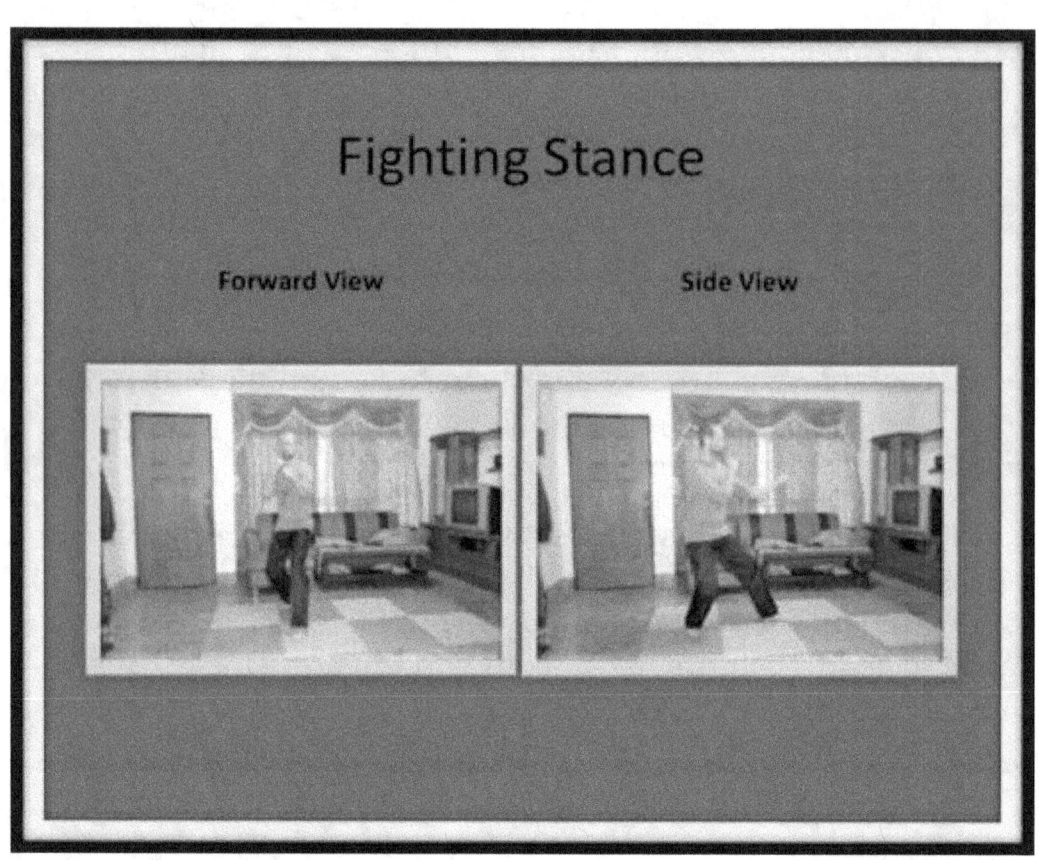

Notes

_____

_____

_____

_____

_____

_____

_____

_____

_____

_____

_____

_____

_____

_____

_____

# Notes

## Unit 4: Blocks

Before learning to punch or kick, the students should know how to block. After they have learned the blocks, it is best to begin with some straight punches when having a regular class. The straight punches are showcased in Unit 5: Strikes.

In counter attacking, a block can be a strike, and a strike, transversely, can be a block. That is a simple truth, but unless you know the difference it is hard to make any kind of distinction

The position to teach an introduction to blocking from easily is horse stance. Get into horse stance and show, in order and with each arm; down block, middle block and rising block. For both down block and rising block you begin by folding one arm with a clenched fist under the opposite elbow. The opposite arm and fist are then placed across the torso with the fist positioned next to the ear.

The fist nearest your ear moves back and across the body stopping over the corresponding knee of the same fist. The opposite fist is placed at the waist on the same corresponding side. The fist should be about two inches away from and directly over the knee. Repeat three times on both sides.

Next, you chamber the one hand under the elbow of the opposite arm directly across the torso. The opposite arm is held in front of the shoulder making a 140° angle at the elbow. Swing the arm held under the elbow out to the same position in front of the shoulder, or in some cases the sternum, with the elbow making a 140° angle. The other hand at this point should pull back to the waist.

Notes

_____

_____

_____

_____

_____

_____

_____

It is not important if the hand is at the shoulder or the sternum at this point. It is only important that you don't over extend the arm by placing it beyond the shoulder. Your blocking power will be decreased, and your risk of hurting your elbow will be increased.

Rising block begins with the hands in the same chambered position as down block. The difference here is that when you release your blocking hand and arm into the block it will be above your head. The arm should be over the temple of the same side, and it should be making that oh so special 140° angle at the elbow.

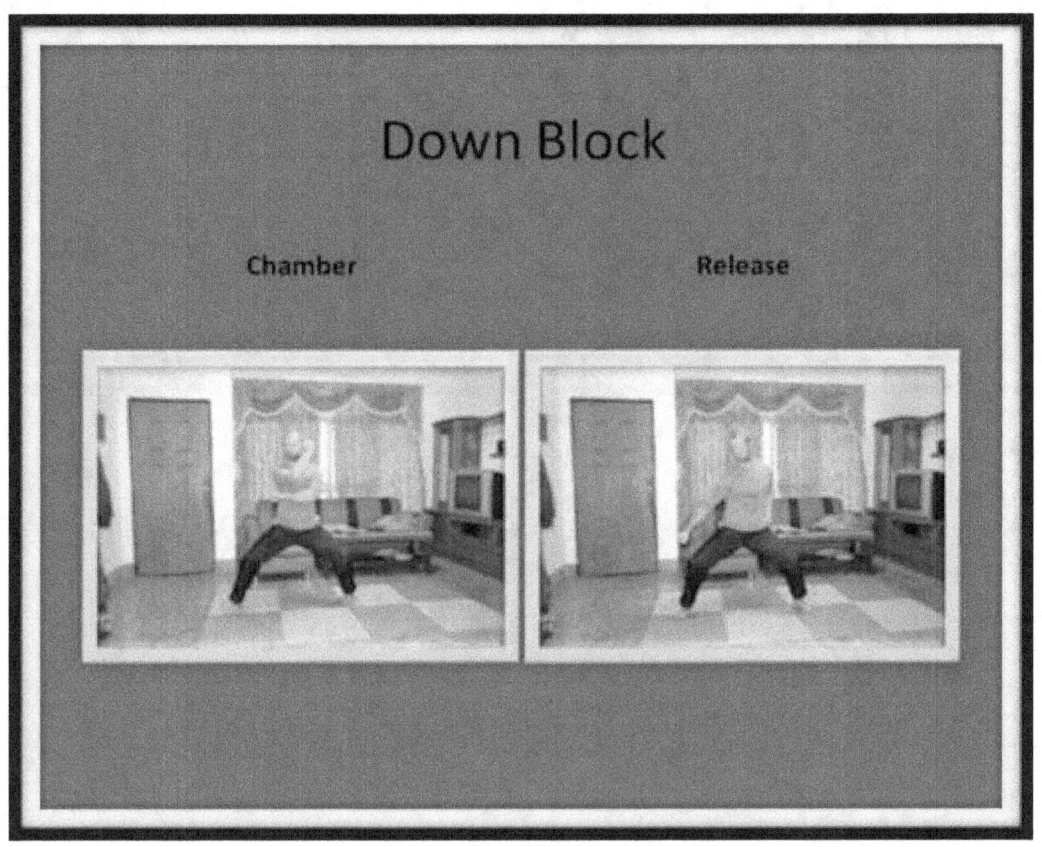

Notes

_____

_____

_____

_____

_____

_____

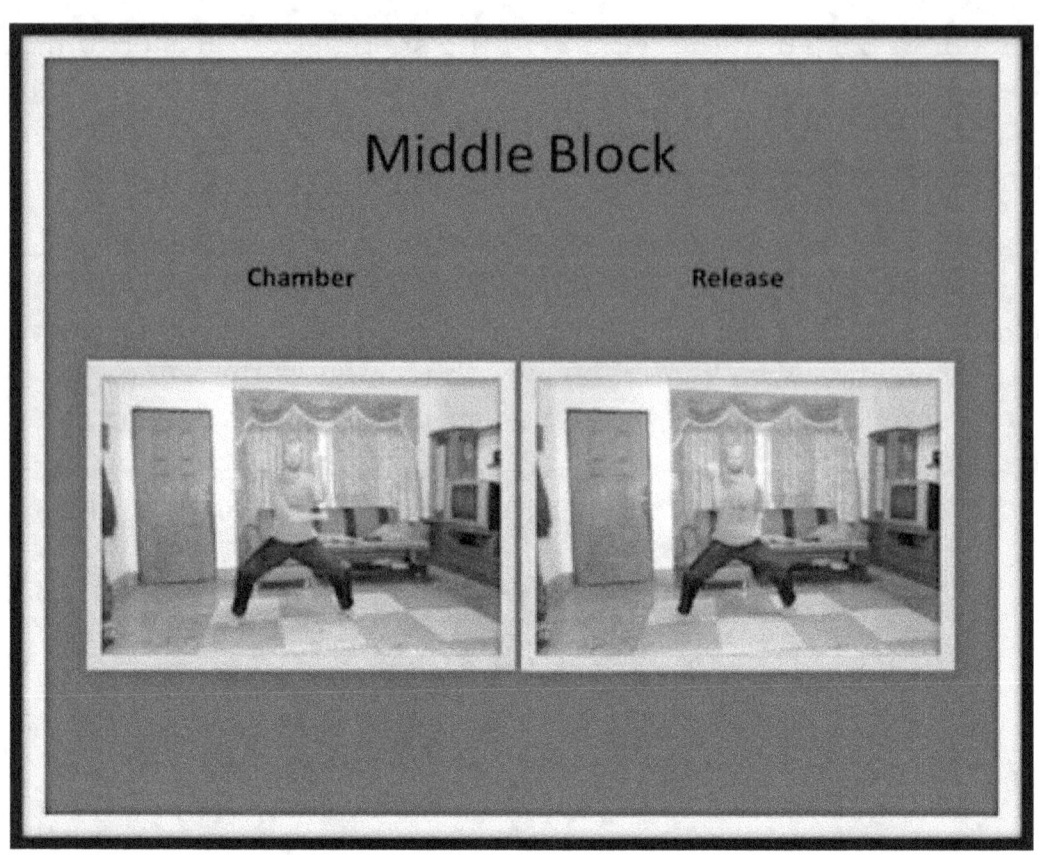

Notes

_____
_____
_____
_____
_____
_____
_____
_____
_____
_____
_____
_____
_____
_____
_____
_____

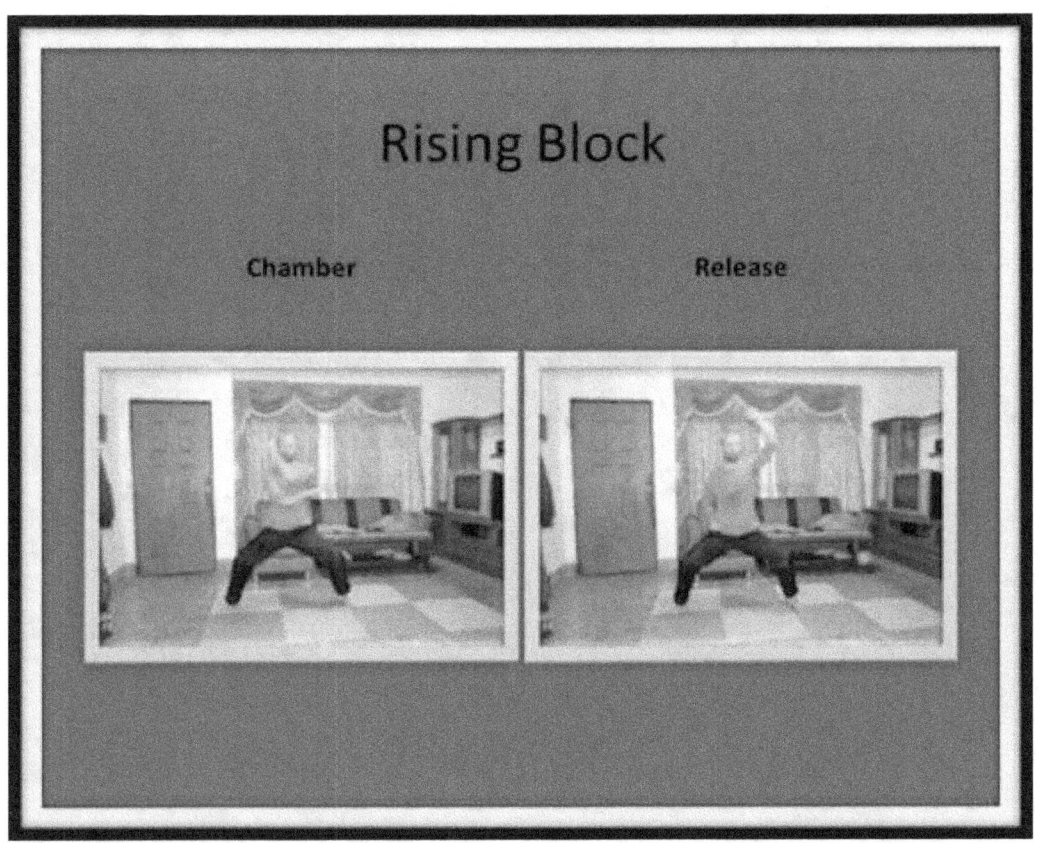

**Rising Block**

Chamber                    Release

Next is pacing and rhythm. Once you have gone through down, middle and rising blocks, you can begin doing block transitions. A good block transition is down on one side, middle on the opposite

side and rising on the same as the down block you started with. You can mix up the transitions as you like, and it is good fun for the kids.

After practicing transitions, double blocking is next on the to do list. First you make an "X" with the forearms in front of your chest. Then throw both arms out over the knees in a double down block. Second, make an "X" between the thighs with your forearms. Throw your arms up into a double middle block. Finally you make an "X" in front of the chest again, and throw your arms up into a double rising block.

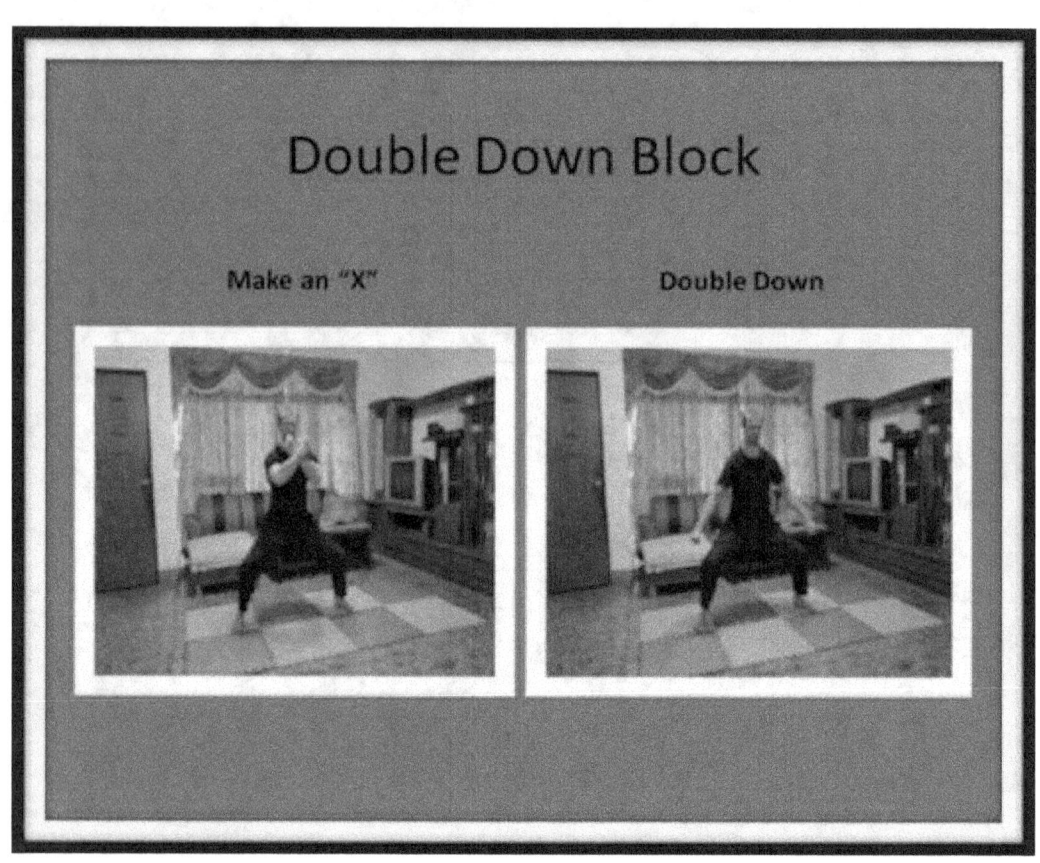

Notes

_____
_____
_____
_____
_____
_____
_____
_____
_____
_____
_____
_____
_____
_____
_____
_____
_____
_____

# Double Middle Block

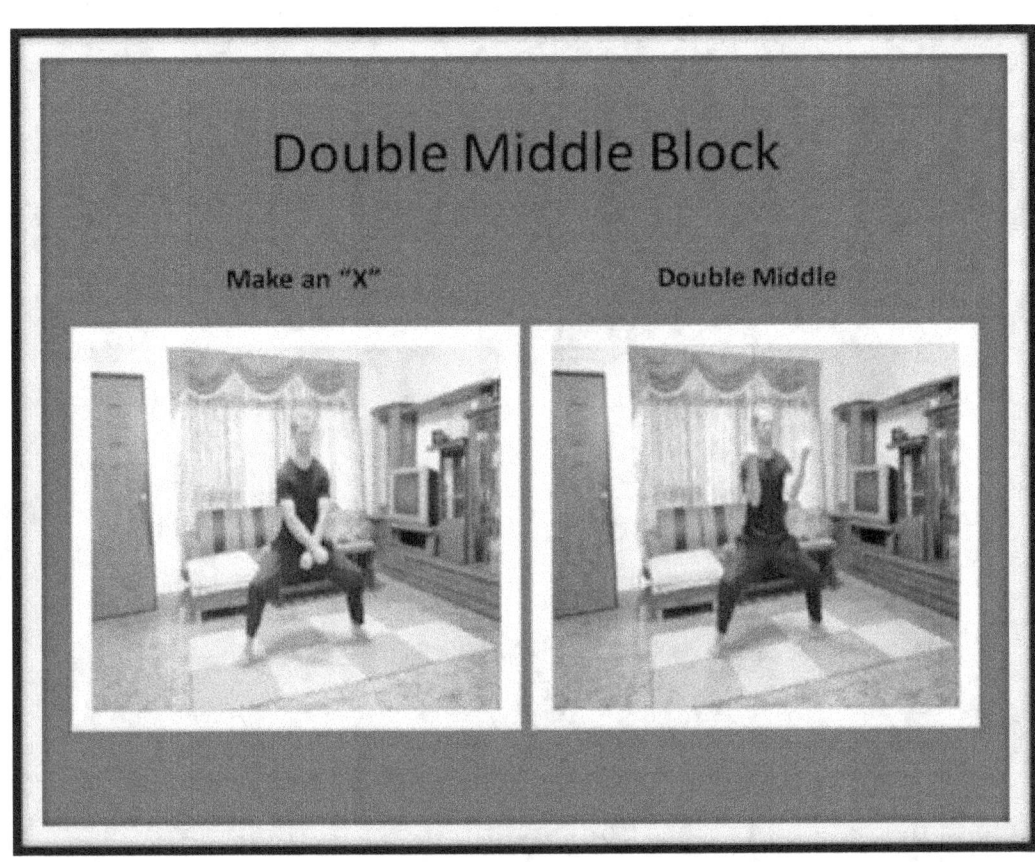

Make an "X"  Double Middle

Notes

_____
_____
_____
_____
_____
_____
_____
_____
_____
_____
_____
_____
_____
_____
_____
_____
_____

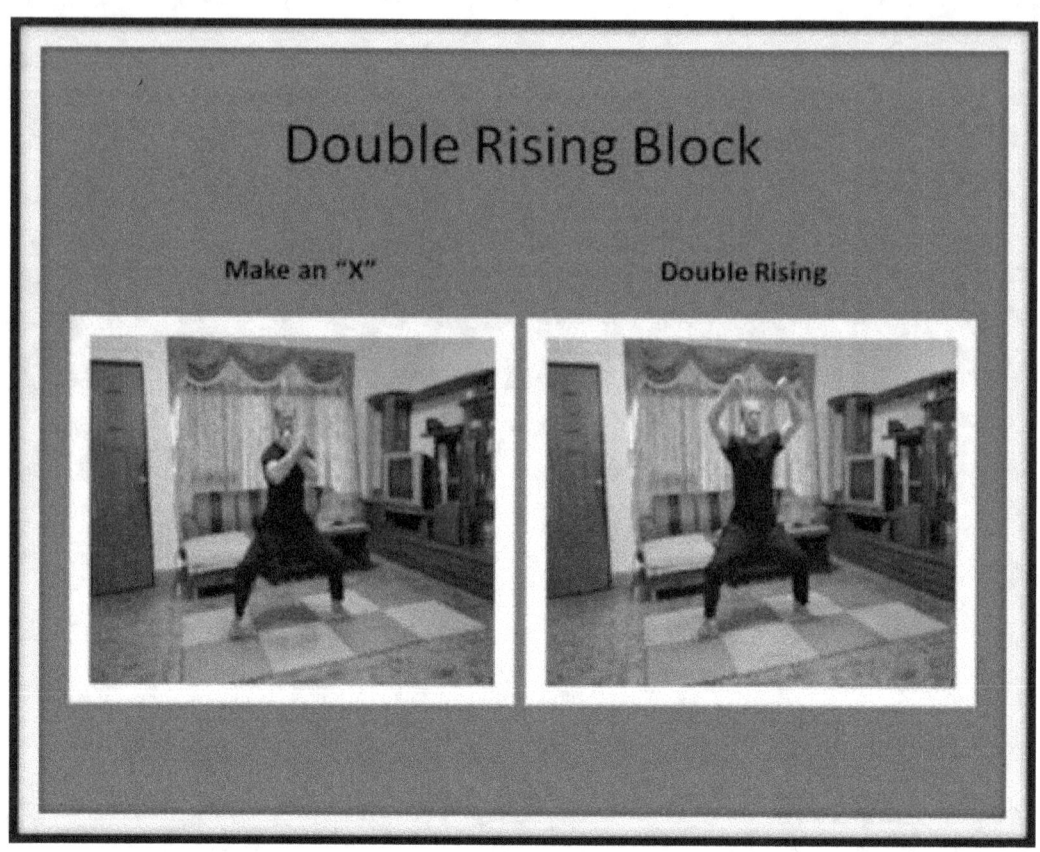

The geometry doesn't need to be pointed out to the kids, ever. Saying one hundred and forty degrees this and ninety degrees that doesn't matter. For them it's more of a see it, do it sort of situation.

And the best they can do is fine, always. In some instances making small corrections is good, but it takes away from the fun of the class. If you make a decent example, overtime they will adapt. You don't have to be perfect of course, but there should be some effort involved.

Notes

_____

_____

_____

_____

_____

_____

_____

# Notes

## Unit 5: Strikes

*Punching*

Beginning in horse stance, the first punch thrown is a simple straight punch. With both fists placed on the waist and facing up, extend one hand out in front of your chest and punch. Do the same thing on the other side while retracting your extended hand back to the waist. The fist of the striking hand should be placed in front of the sternum.

Repeat the same action five or more times, and then punch low. Instead of punching in front of the chest, punch between the thighs a few times. Next, change to striking with the fist just above the head. These punches are referred to as "low, middle and high," punches, and should be done in rhythmic transition much like the blocks.

In transition you can begin by punching low, then to the middle and then high. Use a different arm to strike each time you throw the punches in transition. Then reverse it by going from high to middle and then low. You can change it up and have fun with it in many different ways.

Notes

_____

_____

_____

_____

_____

_____

_____

_____

_____

_____

_____

_____

_____

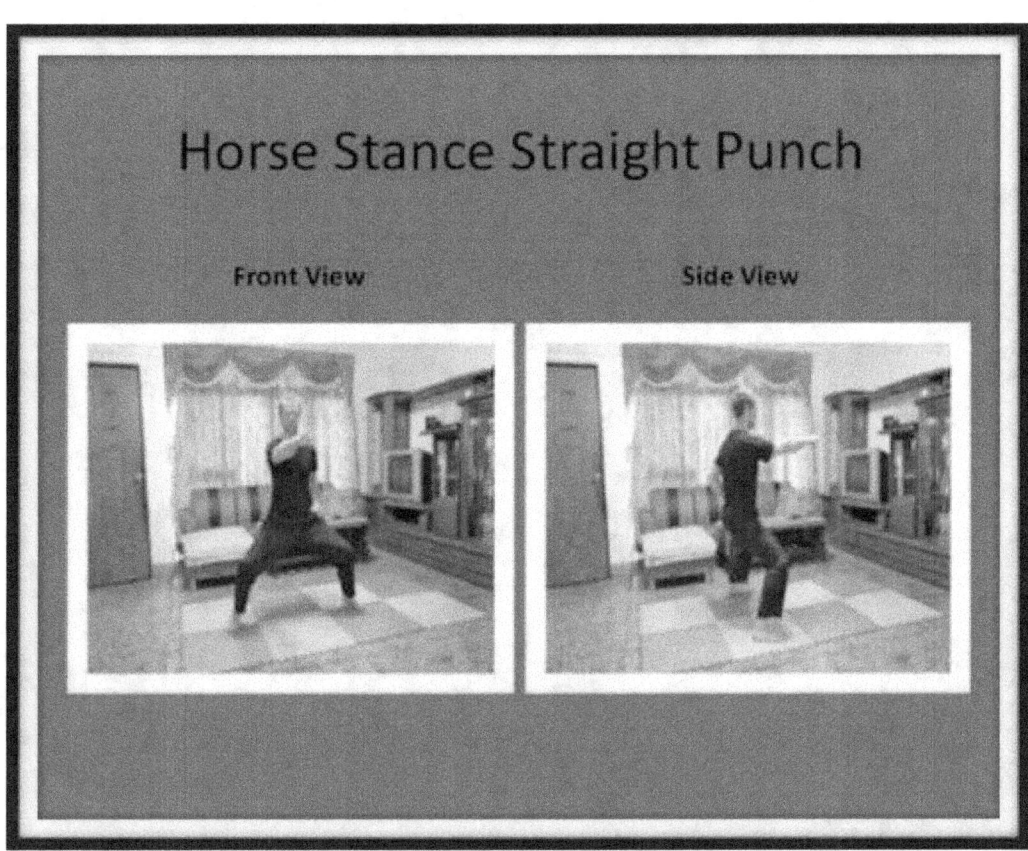

Notes

_____
_____
_____
_____
_____
_____
_____
_____
_____
_____
_____
_____
_____
_____
_____
_____
_____
_____

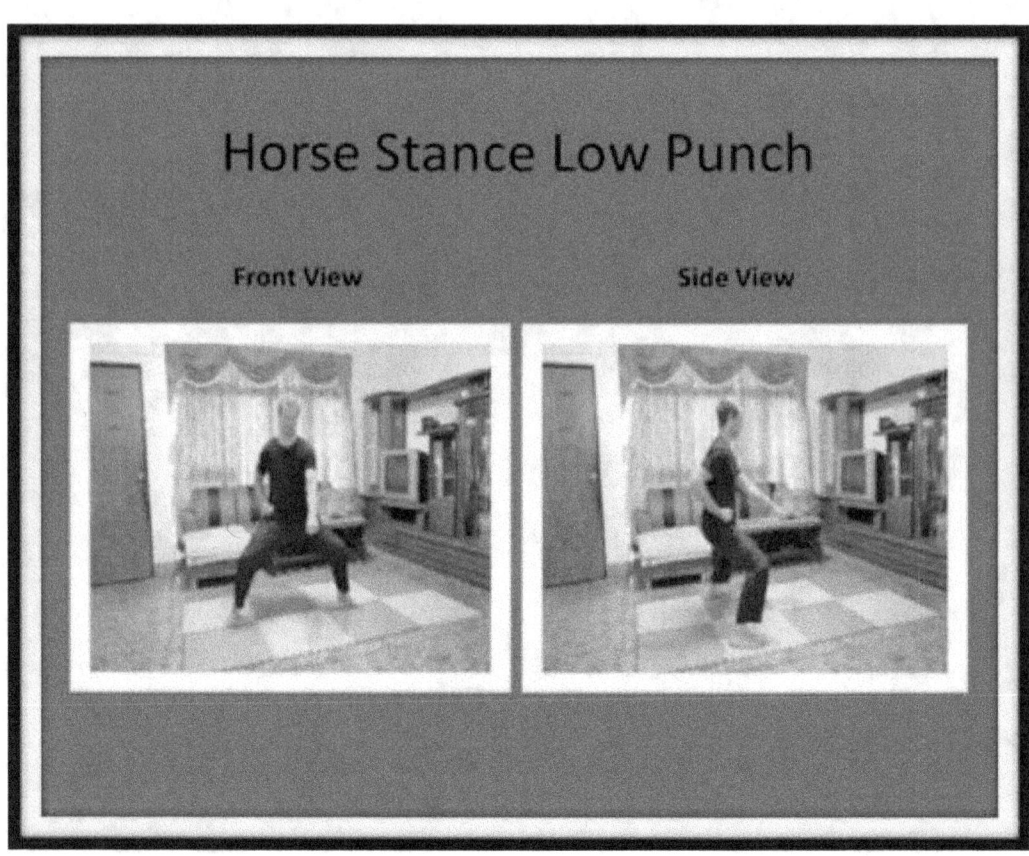

Notes

_____

_____

_____

_____

_____

_____

_____

_____

_____

_____

_____

_____

_____

_____

_____

_____

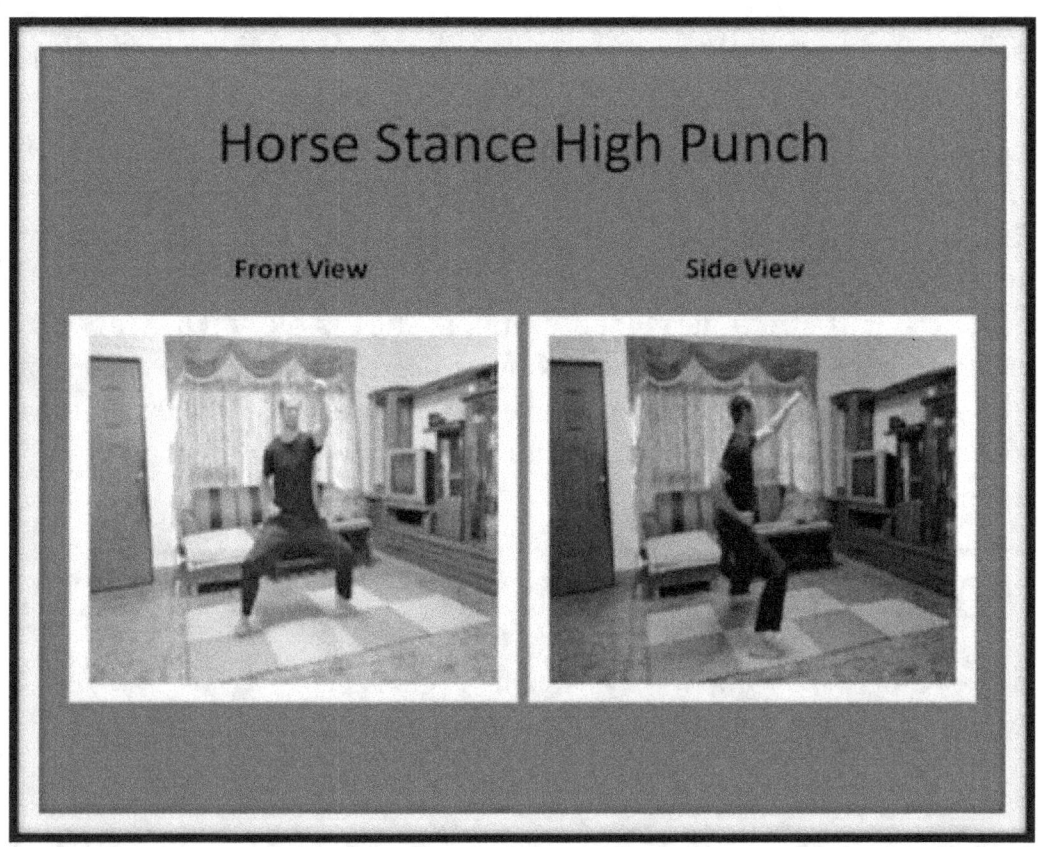

**Horse Stance High Punch**

Front View     Side View

When you finish the segment of horse stance punches, return to ready position. After some time you may switch the order of horse stance punching and blocks in class. I start with horse stance punching, and then blocks before returning to ready position. I usually teach blocks first for a number of classes, and then switch the order. I have found that to be the most effective method for my classes, but it may not work the same way for others.

From ready position, switch into left side forward fighting stance. With the left side forward begin by throwing your front guarding hand straight out at face level. This punch is called a jab. Then retract your front fist and throw out your back hand. This is called reverse.

After displaying the jab and reverse to the kids, do five jabs followed by five reverses. Then do five combinations of jab and reverse. Next, with the back leg bring it up at the knee to waist high saying, "just your knee." Bring the hand on the same side as the leg down to touch the top of the knee. Next repeat the same punches and knees on the right side.

Practicing bringing the knee up is to get the children familiar with the correct starting movement when executing a front kick or roundhouse kick. In the beginning many of the kids will not be using the correct hand to punch, or the right knee to kick. They may not even be in a very good stance. That is okay. Only spend a little time correcting them every once in a while, because they won't be able to enjoy the class if you are always correcting them. It's a process, but in no time they actually pick things up and correct themselves.

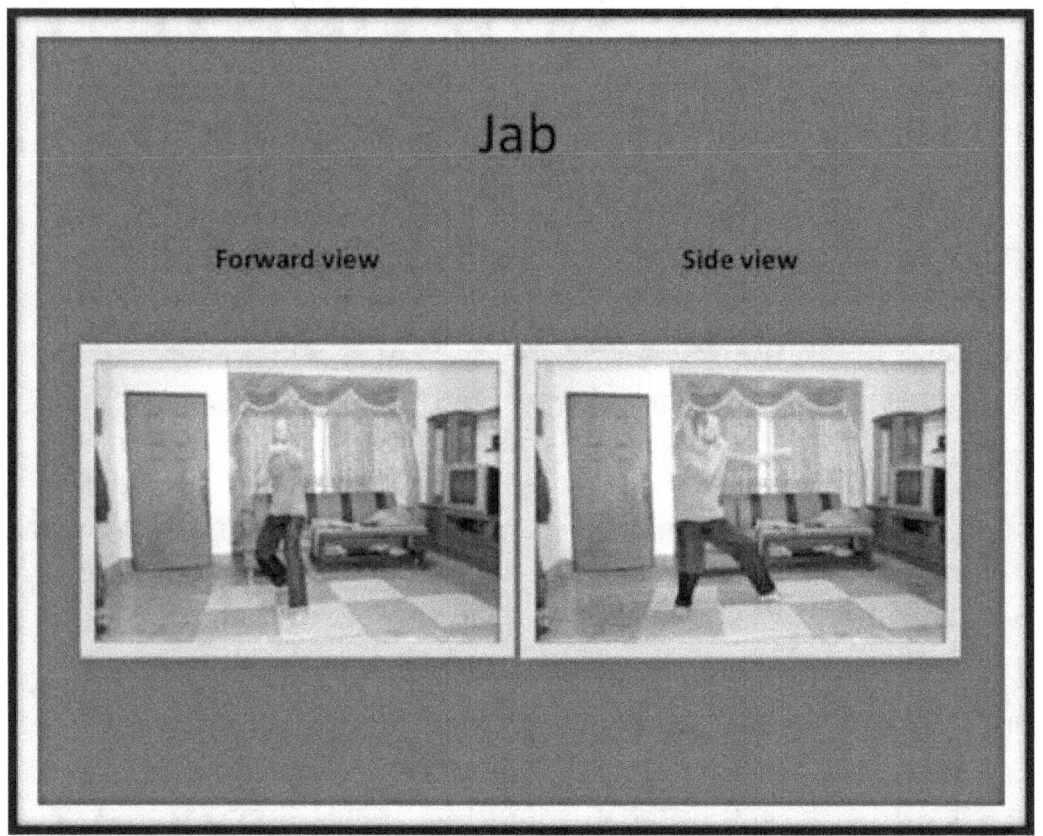

Notes

_____

_____

_____

_____

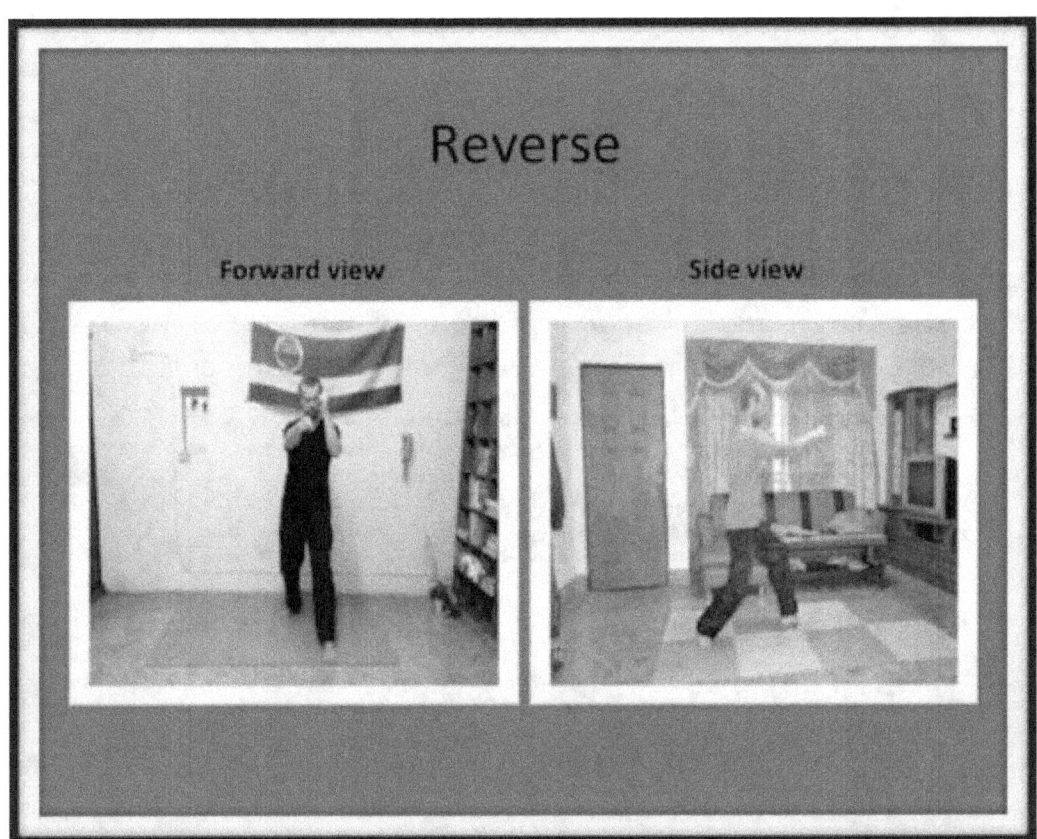

*Kicking*

Once you've practiced in a number of classes (say 8-10) with just bringing the knee up, you can show the kids how to do a front kick. It is the same as bringing the knee up, but you don't lower your hand to touch the top of the knee. Instead, when it is waist high, throw your foot straight out with the toes bent back as when you are practicing the seated hand techniques after lion stretch.

It is important to have the toes pointed back so you can avoid breaking them when striking a target or opponent. Not that you or the kids will be hitting anything, but is necessary to avoid injury and important to perform the techniques appropriately.

Roundhouse kicks are covered in the advanced section, but are essentially the same with a minor adjustment. It is best at this point to reiterate the rules about being nice to others. Generally, I ask the questions about hitting others and when you have a problem at the end of class, but you can ask them whenever you so choose.

This is also a key point at which to monitor that the kids are not too close to one another. They can, by accident, go too far this way or that and hit someone or get hit do to a general lack of balance and control. There will be some that do it on purpose. For both accidents, and the malicious little ones, I put them in timeout for a little bit. I give a longer timeout for the ones who are in fact trying to hurt others, and will increase their punishment accordingly.

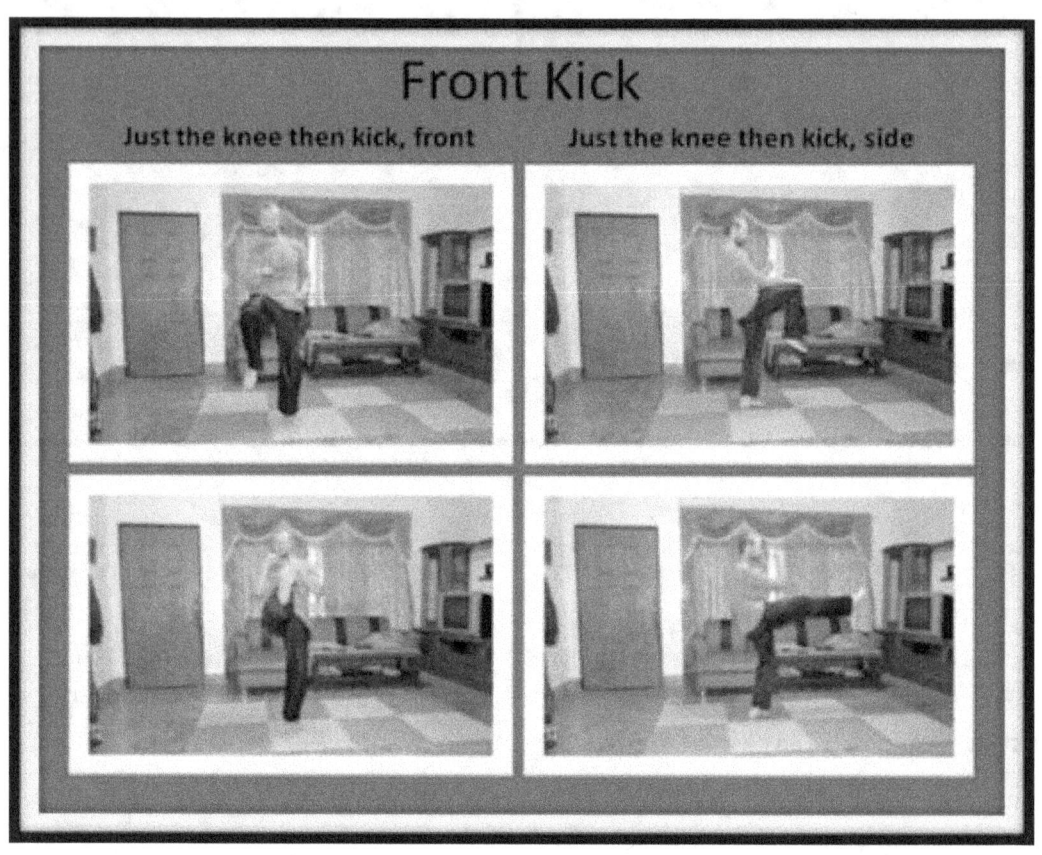

Notes

_____

_____

_____

_____

_____

_____

# Notes

## Unit 6: Rolls, Advanced Techniques and Demonstrations

The advanced material is primarily for children who have already done at least fifty to sixty classes. Generally, I teach the three to four year olds everything but the advanced techniques. I also leave out some of the stretches as I have mentioned. Advanced techniques are more suitable for kids age five to seven or eight.

*+Forwards and Bacwards rolls*

Rolls are by far the most complicated techniques in the book. They are also the most dangerous techniques to teach children in this program if done incorrectly, so it is very important to understand this section well before attempting to teach rolling.

Things you will need:

1.) Mats (puzzle piece, or otherwise)

2.) A large clear path

3.) Patience

You can begin by having the children put one knee down and turned 90°. The other leg should be placed out in front as though you are kneeling to propose or be knighted. You place your hands and arms in a diagonal outward facing circle. The fingertips of the hands should be close to touching one another, about a fingers width apart.

Now place the hands on the ground by the knee of the leg facing out in front of your torso. You should practice having the children hold their hands out in front, and then placing the hands on the ground at least three or four times to make sure they understand thoroughly. You may need at this point to physically correct the position of some of the students.

When you roll, you roll from the shoulder of the leg facing out in front through to the hip of the opposite side. It is a good idea to illustrate this for the children. You can do so by holding a rope or the handle of a broom or mop across your back from your shoulder to the hip on the opposite side of the body.

Be sure to look at the pictures titled front rolls. I seldom if ever teach backward rolls to the students, but I do demonstrate the rolls so they are also included in the pictures. If you have a class of students that is particularly good at front rolls, I recommend teaching the back rolls. Otherwise, I wouldn't suggest it.

In a backwards roll you sort of sit back placing your hands down for support behind you. Then you roll across the back from the hip of the rear leg to the shoulder on the opposite side kicking front leg up. The front leg will be the first part that comes back up as you finish the roll.

Pointing out that you do not hit the ground with your head at any time is imperative. It is something they should already be familiar with from learning the seated back and side falls. You can demonstrate this by telling the students to watch you. Go down as if you are going to place your head on the ground first, but stop. Ask the children, "Should you hit the ground with your head?"

When you get to the end of the roll you should be back in the same position where you began. At the beginning, the students will, for the most part, be unable to do anything more than roll on their sides. There will most likely be a few stand outs that can understand the concepts and apply the physics. Don't stress over their performances. Point out the students that are good, but make sure the others have their turn and enjoy their time.

With both rolls and front falls, I stop the regular class after stretching. For rolls and front falls, you need time, space and you have to set up the mats. I have the children sit on the colored tape and practice getting into the right position. When they are ready I will usually bring up two students at a time to practice front falls, and one student at a time to practice rolls.

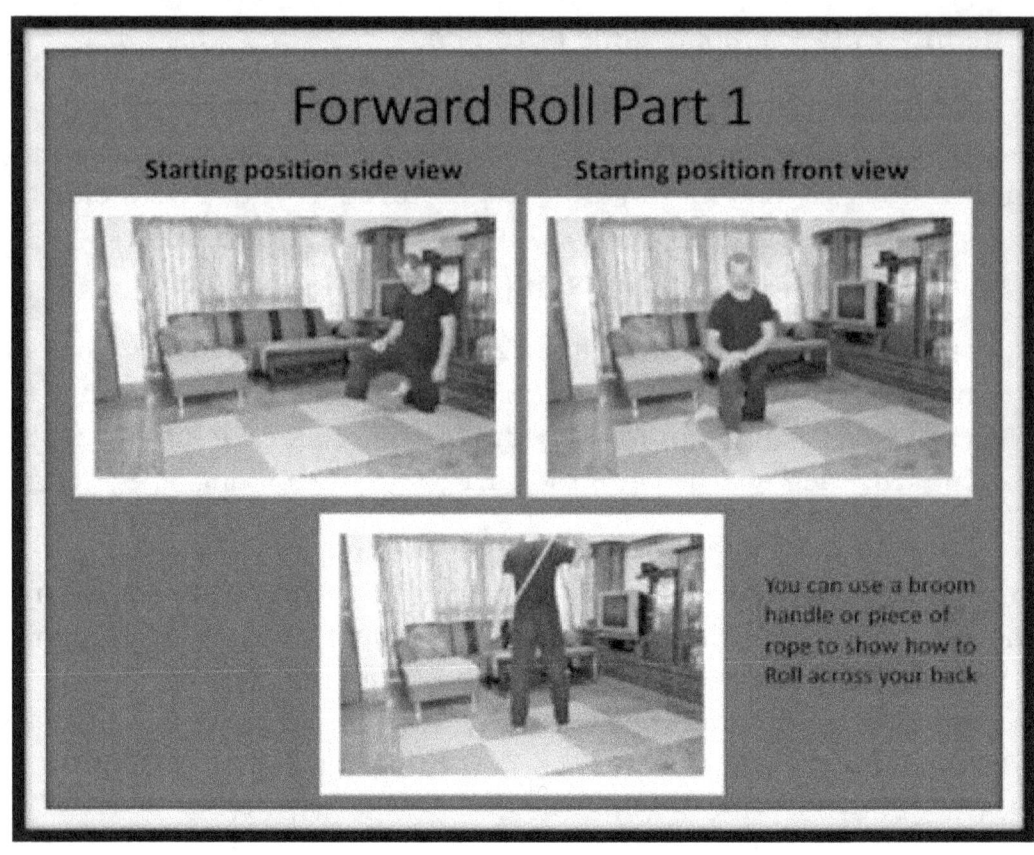

Notes

_____

_____

_____

_____

_____

_____

_____

_____

_____

_____

_____

_____

_____

_____

_____

_____

_____

_____

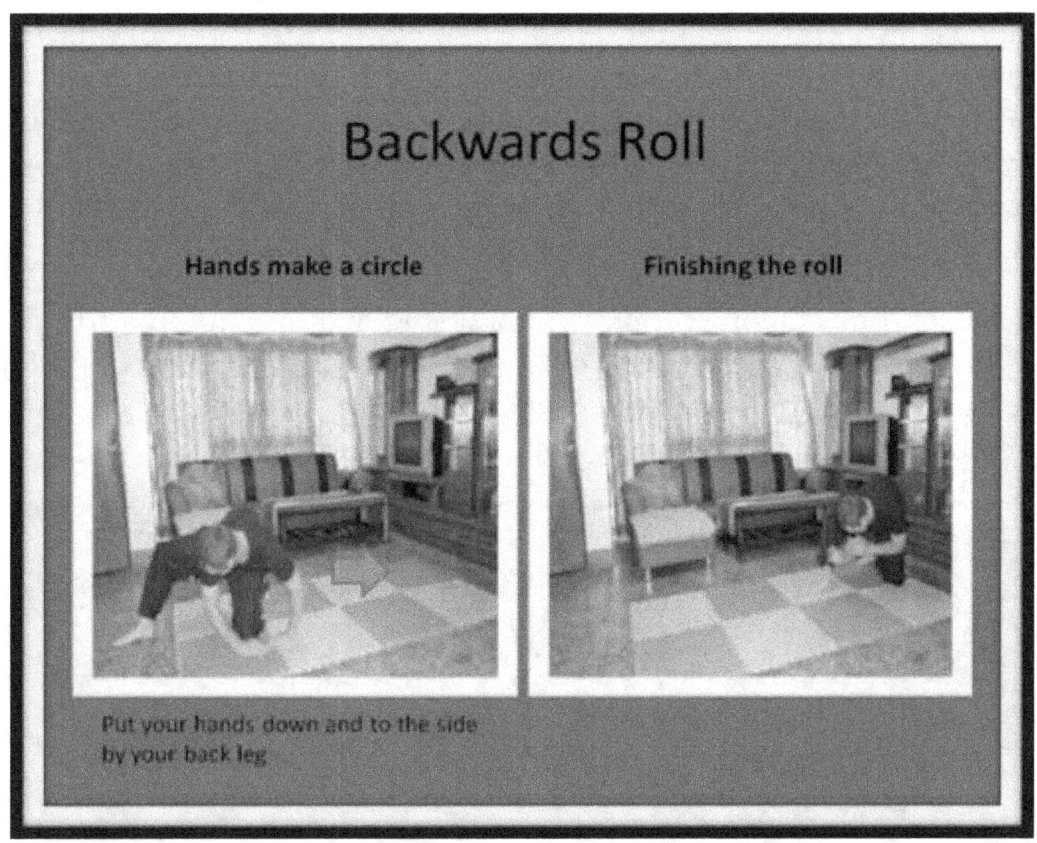

*+Advanced Seated Hand Techniques*

After the children have gotten a little bit older they can begin learning two more seated techniques. They will be able to sit on their knees for longer, and will be capable of understanding more complex movements. All seated techniques begin with the fingertips rising like a paintbrush stroking the tops of the legs, and the hands coming up in front of your torso.

Notes

The next two seated techniques are as follows. First, the hands move out and away from each other with the palms facing down. The hands come back to cross each other with the palms facing in towards the face. Let the hands then move down towards the center of the knees, and the hand closest to the face goes back to your ear.

The second movement consists of pressing with one hand and pulling with the other. Then you abruptly change the direction of the hands with the hand which was pulling, pushing in and up. The hand which was pressing will pull out and down.

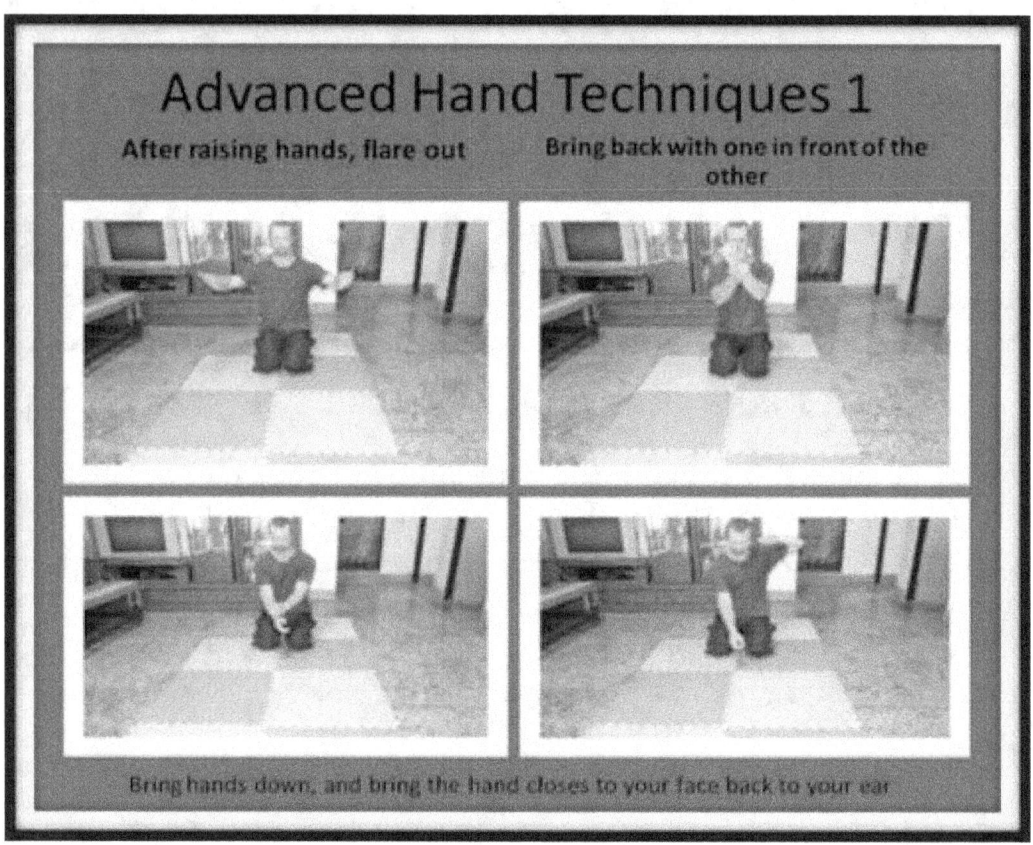

Notes

_____

_____

_____

_____

_____

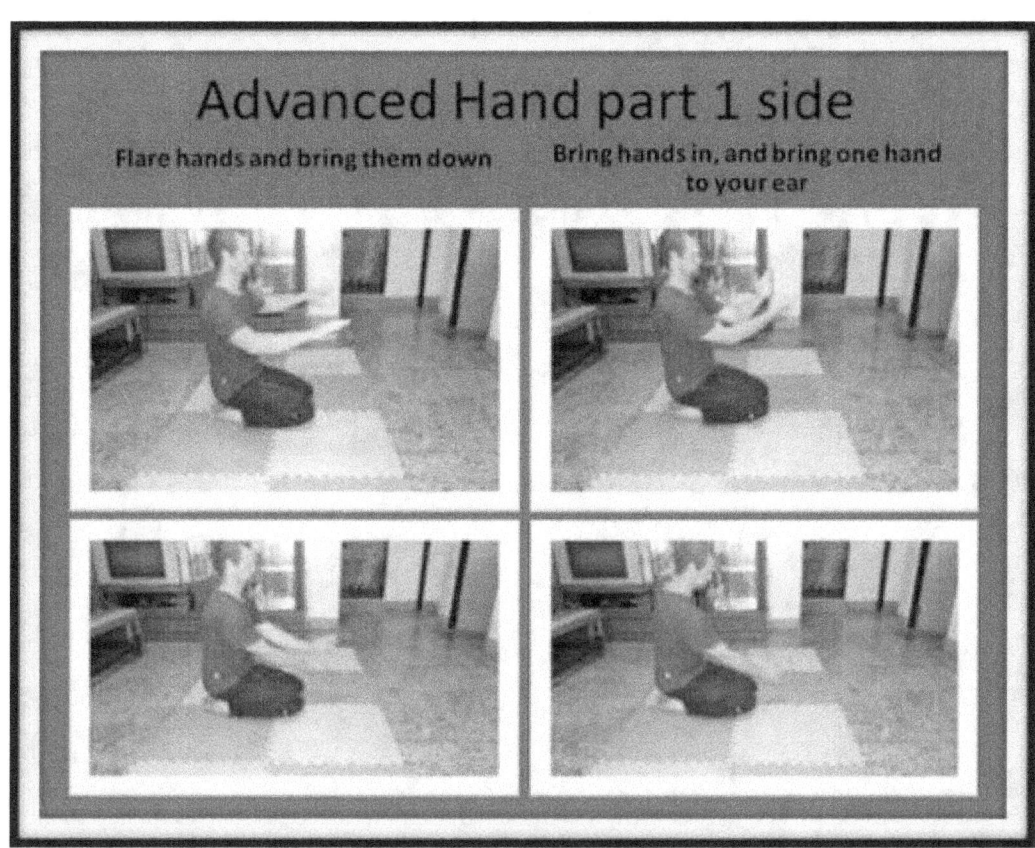

Notes

_____

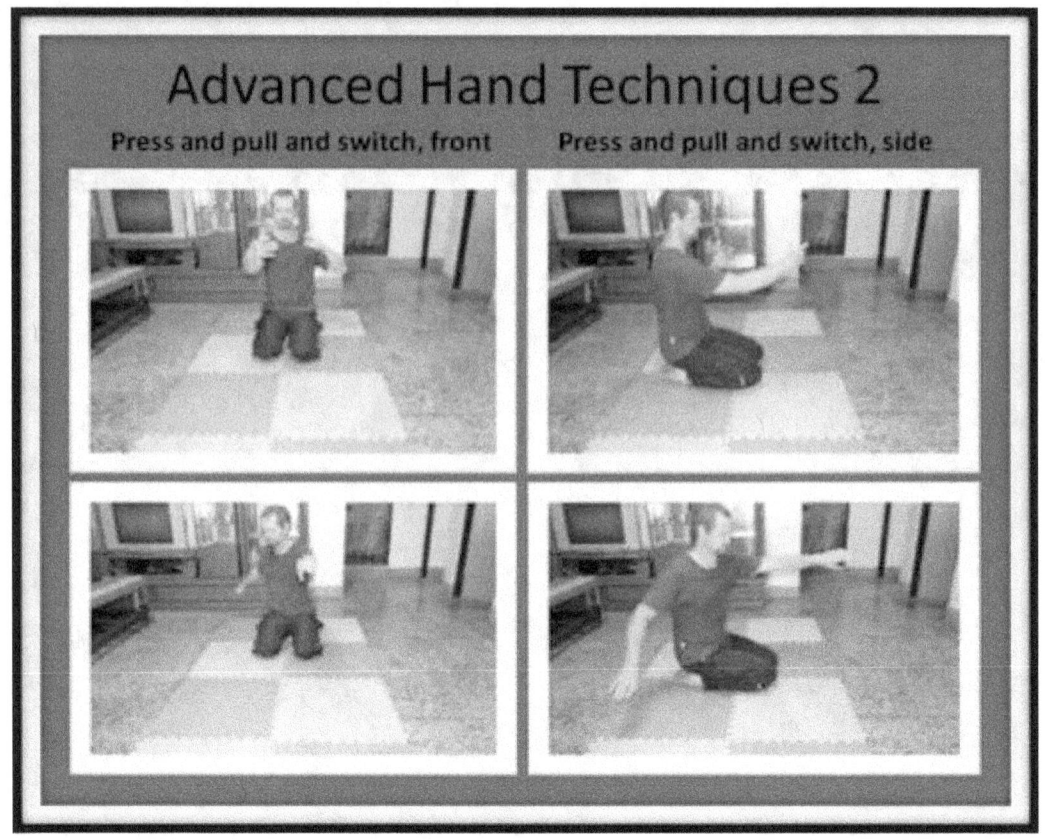

**Advanced Hand Techniques 2**

Press and pull and switch, front     Press and pull and switch, side

+*Advanced kicking: Roundhouse kick*

As you continue to learn the material with the kids, you may wish to include more techniques. If you wish to go beyond the advanced material that I have outlined here, I would recommend first letting the children decide if they are truly interested in martial arts all that much. My goal is to give the kids a small example and a few things which can help them protect themselves from injury while developing a non-violent attitude.

With that said, it wouldn't hurt to include a side kick or crescent kick. If a child is truly interested in learning more, I would recommend finding a martial arts school.

A roundhouse kick is a simple transition from front kick. As you are practicing seated hand techniques you learn to sit on your toes, and then you change your feet to have the instep facing the floor. With the toes curled up, you learn the proper way to execute a front kick or front snap kick. The feet, with the instep facing down, is the proper way to execute a roundhouse kick.

As with the front kick, you first bring the knee up for the roundhouse. Next turn the hip over as you extend the foot. The foot will act almost like a hand slapping a target, as you strike with the instep of the foot.

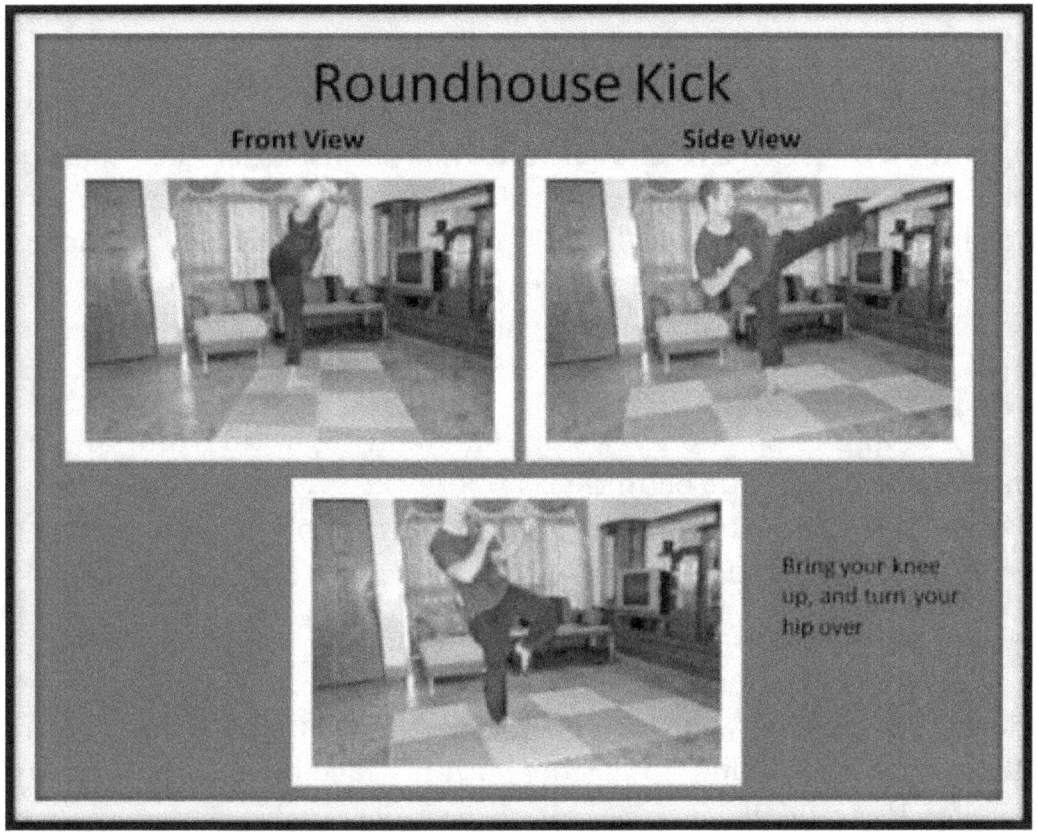

+*Advanced Front Fall*

The front fall, along with rolling, can be a dangerous technique when not performed correctly. You will need mats to execute the front fall properly. You begin by sitting on your knees with the feet flat behind you, as in the second part of the seated hand techniques. When you fall forward you should hit the ground with your hands and forearms.

First demonstrate the front fall by coming forward gently and placing your hands and forearms in a partial triangle shape with your body over the arms. You should not be too far forward or too far back. You can hurt your shoulder if you are not centered well over your forearms.

Have the children slowly repeat your demonstration. It is important not to demonstrate the front fall entirely here, because without the proper precautions there could be injuries. Once you have practiced, probably for one class, gently getting into the proper position, you can perform an actual front fall from the seated position.

When the children have shown that they understand the technique, it is time to demonstrate the front fall. You begin by coming up on your knees and bring your hands up in a similar motion to the paintbrush technique from the seated wrist grips section. Now drop forward and plant your weight on your forearms and hands in a triangle.

From a standing position you can demonstrate a full front fall. Your legs will kick out behind you and form the base of your triangle, while your hands for the top. If you only wish to show the seated front fall, that is fine.

Once again, be sure to talk to the students about falling properly. A good way is of course to demonstrate the wrong way to fall in a safe way by placing your face on the mat. Ask them, "Should you fall on your face?" I like to do this with my face down first, because it makes them laugh.

Notes

_____

_____

_____

_____

_____

_____

_____

_____

_____

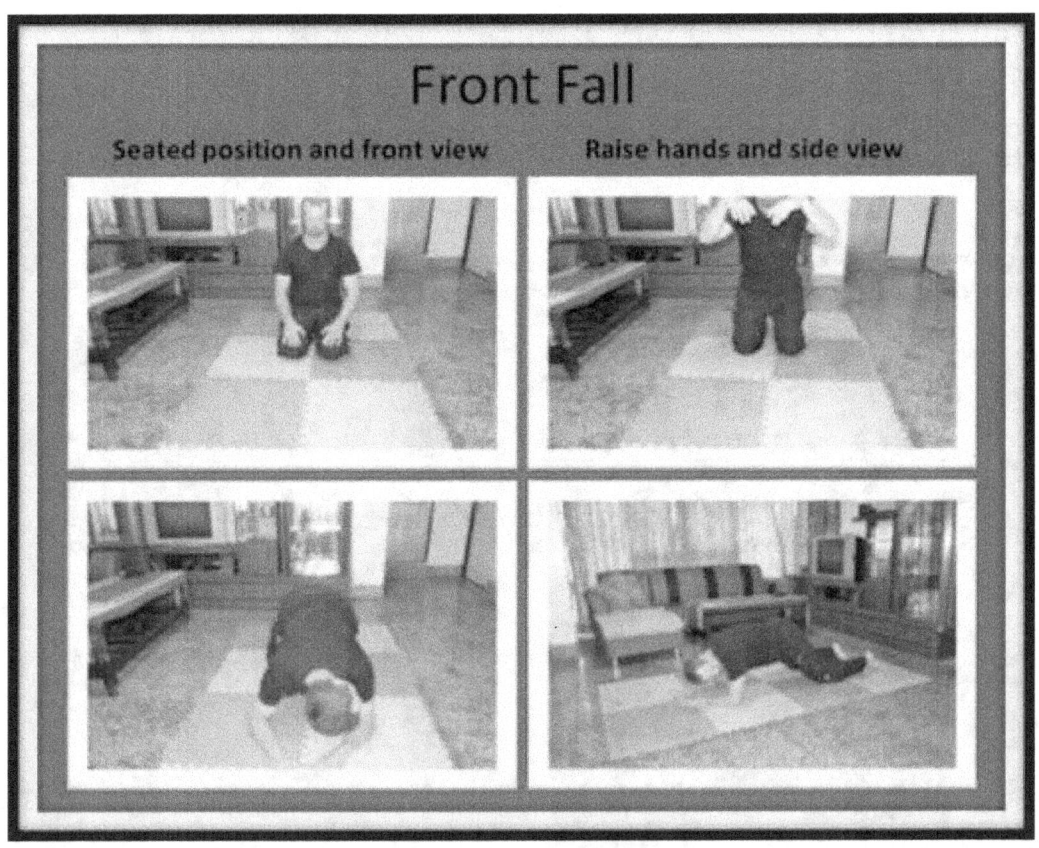

*Front Fall*

Seated position and front view — Raise hands and side view

*+Advanced stances: Front Stance*

Front stance, which is sometimes called archer stance, is performed to a degree in the stretching section already. A major difference between the stretching posture and the actual stance is the placement of the feet. When you are stretching the feet are in a direct line with each other. In front stance, you want your feet to be shoulder width apart.

Starting from ready position, you simply step forward with one leg. The forward leg takes a pretty large step, and about 70% of your weight will rest on the forward leg. Bring your hands up in front of the shoulders with your fists clenched. Practice alternating between the left and right leg, each time returning to ready position to do so.

Front Stance is another opportunity to switch back and forth between ready position and other stances. You could switch to front stance, then fighting stance, and horse stance. Whatever might be fun for the kids is great when transitioning between stances.

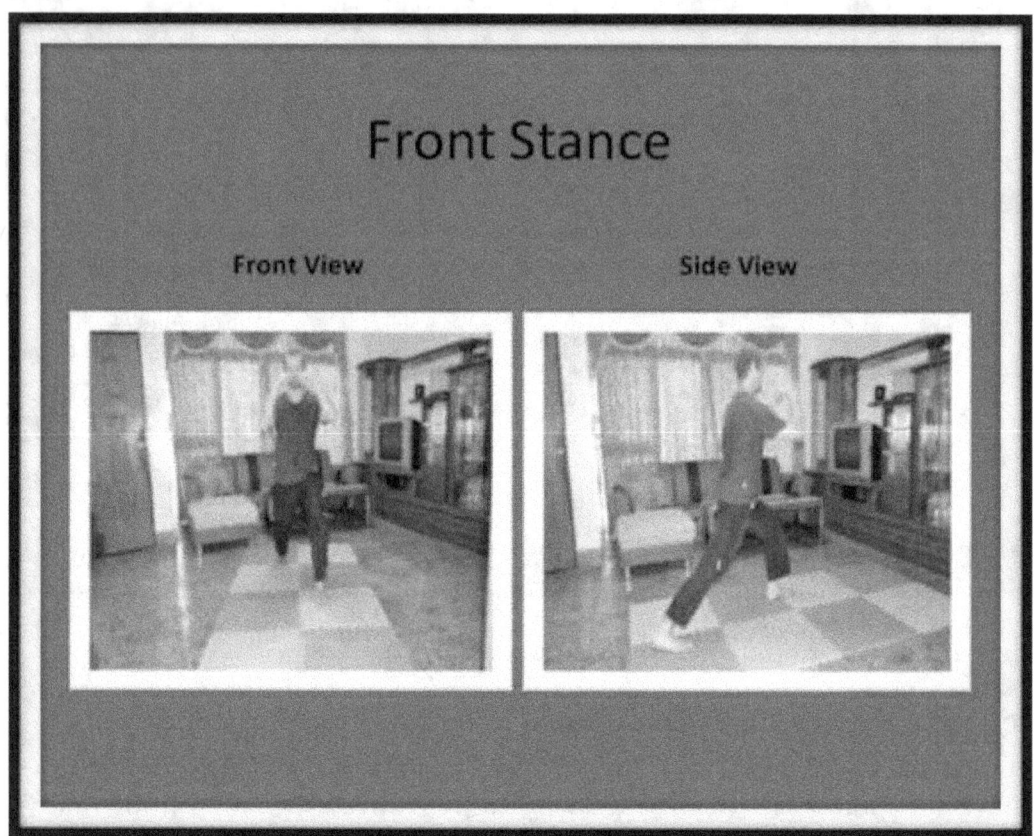

*+Advanced Breathing Techniques*

These breathing techniques are taken from the internal martial arts. They can be referred to as qi gong or yoga. They are good for cooling down at the end of a class, and can easily be taught to younger and older students. The older students will of course gain the greatest benefit from the exercises, because they will understand them better.

Place your feet together as though you are standing at attention. Put the hands on the legs where they naturally fall. Lift the left foot at the heel and step out to shoulders width apart touching the toe down first and then placing the heel down. Sink your weight down into your hips by bending your knees as you start to bring your hands up.

As your hands rise, you can straighten your legs. The hands should only come to about shoulder high, and they should hang very loosely as though you are a marionette with strings at the wrists and elbows. At shoulder high start to let the hands and arms fall back down, and sink your weight back down.

You control your breathing as you do this. Breathe in as your hands come up. Exhale when your hands go down. You can practice stepping out to shoulder width and back to feet together each time before you raise your hands and arms.

## Notes

_____

_____

_____

_____

_____

_____

_____

_____

_____

_____

_____

_____

_____

_____

_____

_____

_____

_____

_____

_____

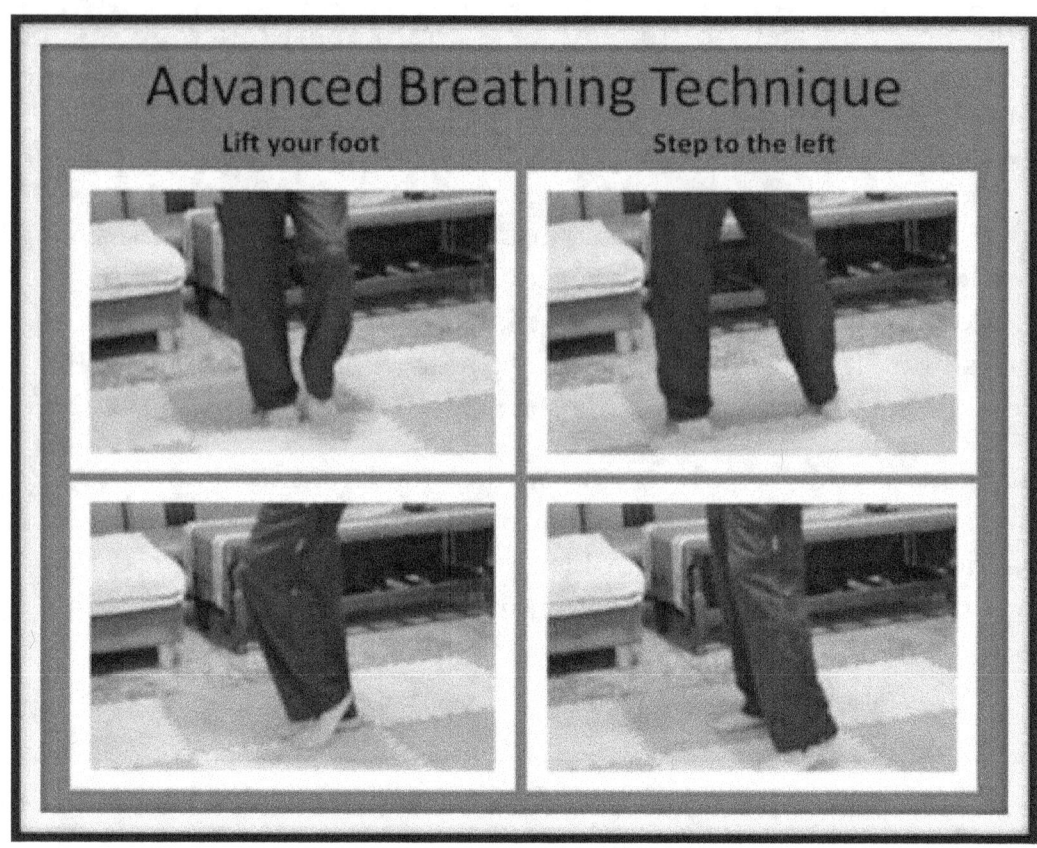

**Advanced Breathing Technique**

Lift your foot          Step to the left

Notes

_____
_____
_____
_____
_____
_____
_____
_____
_____
_____
_____
_____
_____
_____
_____

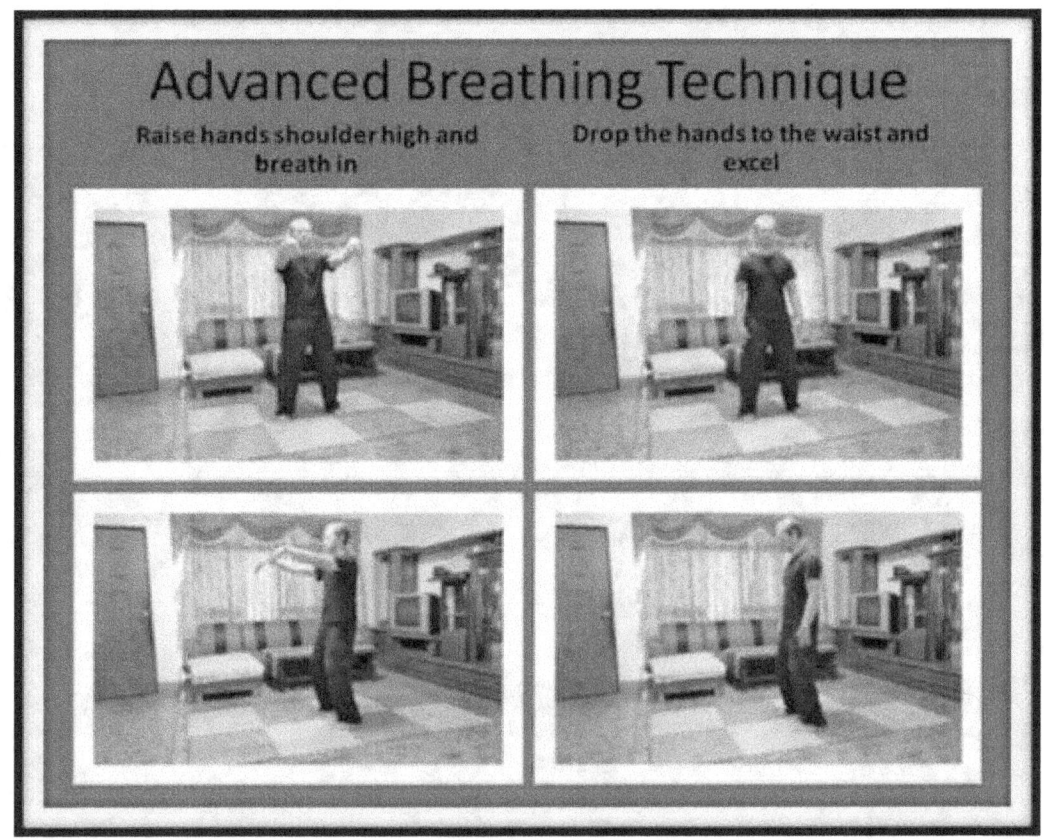

*+Advanced Stretching*

The pictures from the advanced stretching techniques are included here. For the most part the pictures are self-explanatory, but they have been explained in the stretching section. Please refer back to stretching for details.

Notes

_____
_____
_____
_____
_____
_____
_____
_____
_____
_____

# Hamstring Stretch

**Left Leg**

**Right Leg**

Say, "touch your ankle, and if you can touch your ankle, try to touch your toes"

Notes

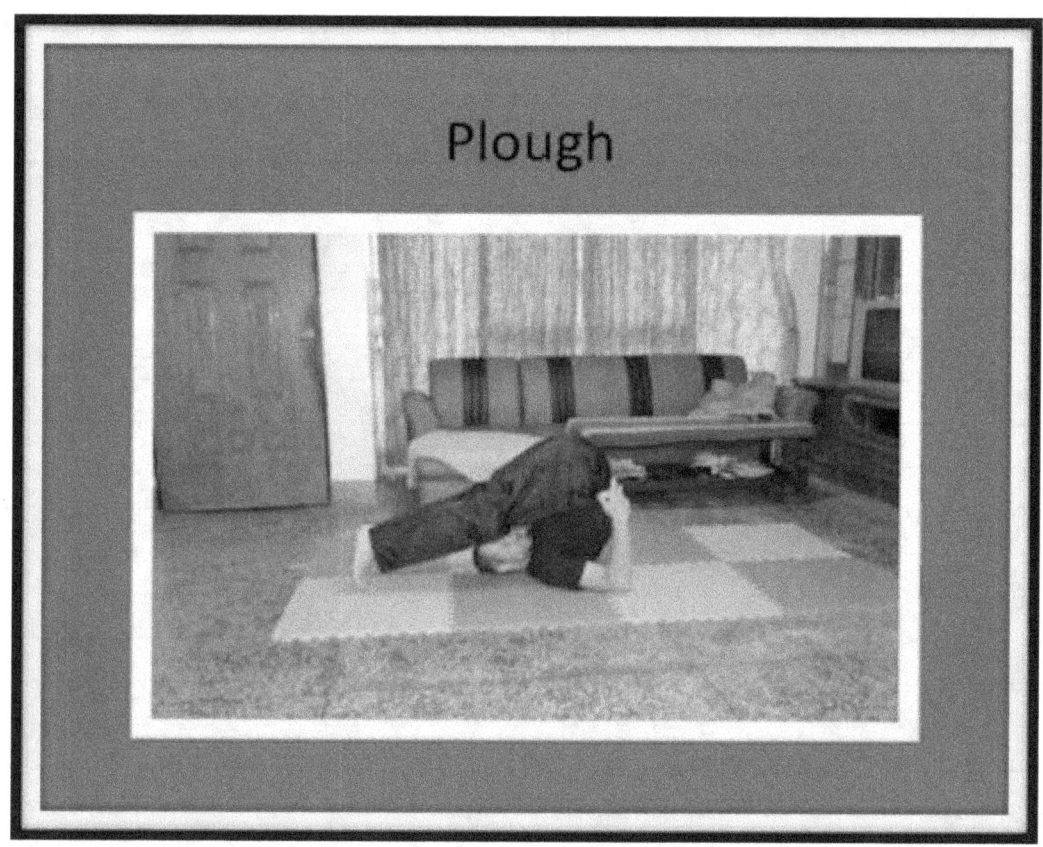

Plough

*+Demonstrations*

If you have already studied martial arts, it would be a good idea to prepare a small demonstration of what martial arts is at the beginning of the first class. You might do so by showing a kata or form, or possibly some kicking techniques that the children probably won't learn in class. It makes them excited for the class, and even if you aren't teaching the material they will be happier practicing after seeing your performance.

If you haven't been studying martial arts prior to beginning this course, you could possibly prepare a video for the children to watch on an Ipad, laptop, TV or other viewing device. Here is a link to me performing a kata (known as "poomse" in Korean) called Goreo from the Korean style of Tae Kwon Do: http://www.youtube.com/watch?v=ysN3w2zzBMY

# Notes

## Unit 7 Games, Closing Statements and Class Flow Chart

*+Games*

As I mentioned before, it may not always be necessary to talk to the class about behavior and the way they should treat others. Often, the students will be well behaved and do some good work in the class. On those occasions it is a good idea to play a game.

The game that seems to be the easiest to play without needing any extra materials is called "four corners," or "go, go, go." It's really simple. You choose four corners of the room and give each a name such as corner number 1, hamburger corner or something else. Then you close your eyes and say go, go, go. If you call corner number 2, and there are children in that corner they are out and have to sit back down on the colored tape.

Whoever is the last one standing can call out in the next game, or you can give them a prize. It is best, once the kids understand the game, to change the names of the corners to add interest to the game and make it seem fresh.

Other games that you might play for the last little bit of a class are; teacher says (sometimes called Simon says); duck, duck goose; musical chairs (if you have the right chairs). Games should be seen as a reward for good behavior. Be sure to remind your students at the beginning of some classes that there might be a game if they are good, and it should help the classes go more smoothly.

*+closing statements*

I have seen many positive results from developing the class. The kids are much better at protecting themselves on the playground as a result of learning how to fall properly. Their general balance and flexibility has also shown vast improvement. The class also helps to curb aggressive behavior.

The key to a successful Kindie Kung Fu class is knowing the material well. If you know what you are doing from beginning to end, then the children will see how confident you are. They will in turn feel confident themselves, which is good but can be dangerous. Be careful with overly confident children.

With everything in the class, from the simplest stretching technique to the advanced rolling, the best your students can do is as good as it gets. Don't try to force perfection on the kids, because they won't have fun if you do. I know this from personal experience. Make sure to correct bad behavior within the grounds of good taste, but let them have fun.

As you progress with teaching and learning the material yourself, you can see what works and how to make a more cohesive class. It is a process, and may take some time to really get the kinks out. When it is working well, and the kids are having fun in a safe way, every effort is worth the end result. I wish you the best of luck in your endeavor to learn, teach and understand the material.

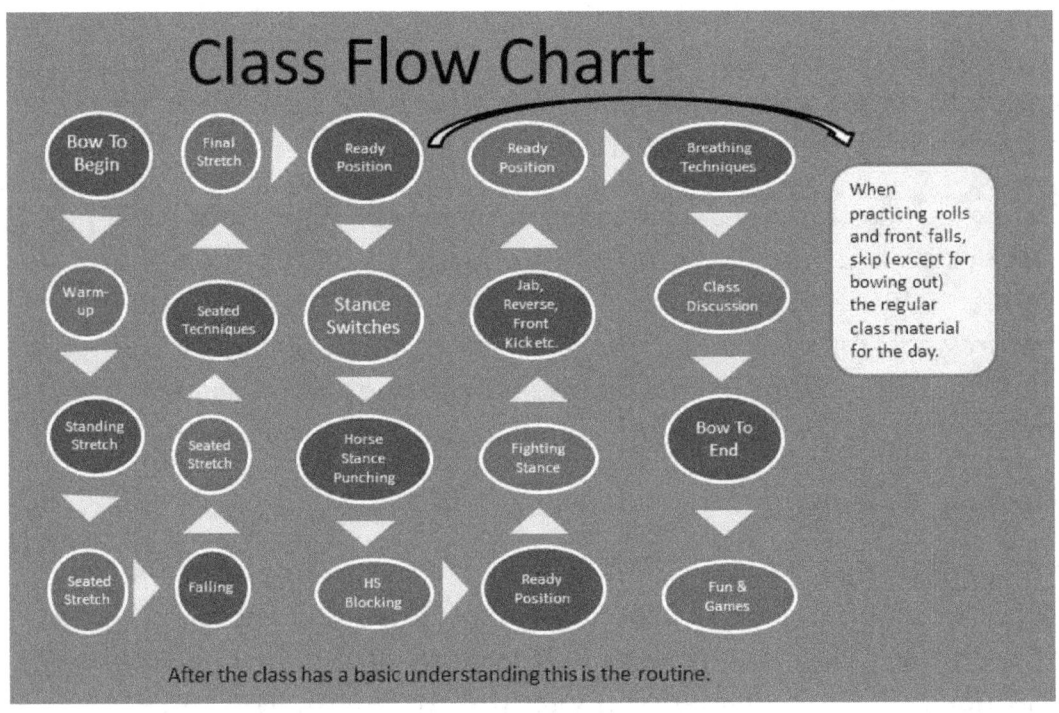

***The End***

Connect online here:

https://www.facebook.com/KindieKungFu

# Notes

# Notes

# Notes

# Notes

**Connect Online**

https://www.facebook.com/KindieKungFu

https://sites.google.com/site/kindiekungfu/

https://plus.google.com/u/0/b/114673986577967742019/114673986577967742019/posts

**Other Books By the Author**

Selected Poetry And Songs

Kindie Kung Fu (in Spanish)

Hiragami's Box

**Coming Soon**

Nitwits, Nimrods and Nincompoops; Semi-autobiographical Tales of the Befuddlingly Inane

With Prejudice

Three Ranges Boxing

To purchase this book or other books by William Gentry go to Createspace.com or Amazon.com and search for William Gentry and / or titles of books from above